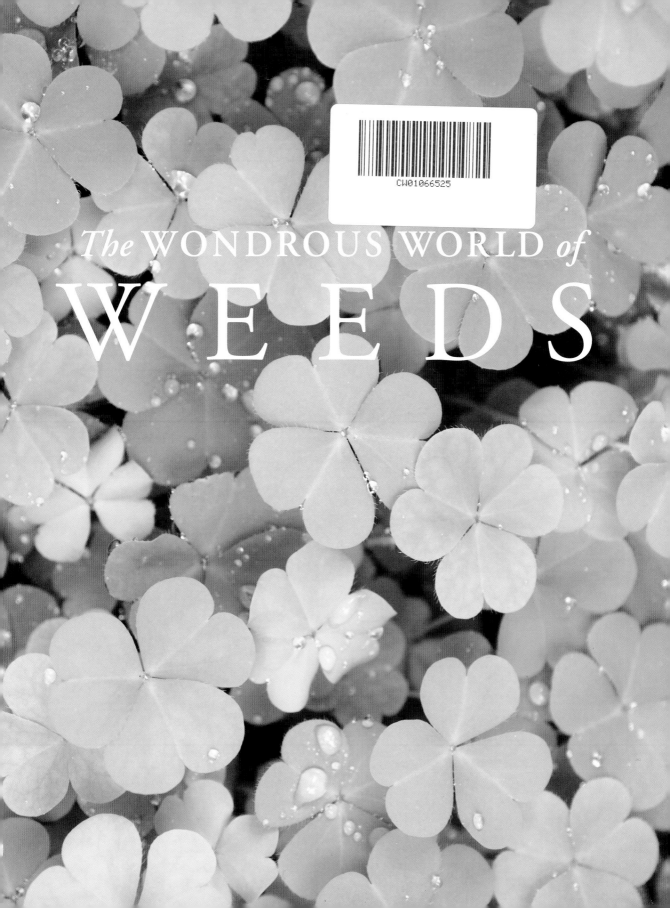

The WONDROUS WORLD of
WEEDS

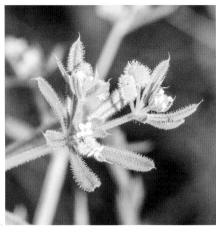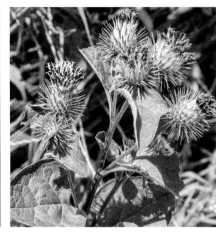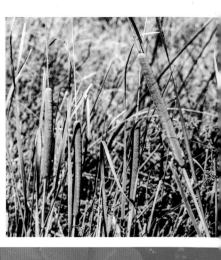

The WONDROUS WORLD of

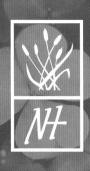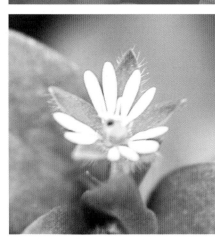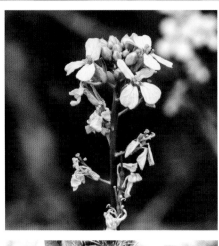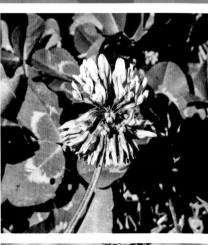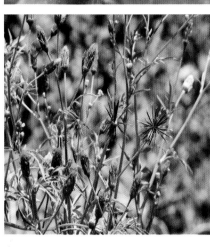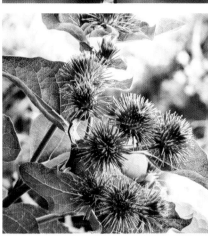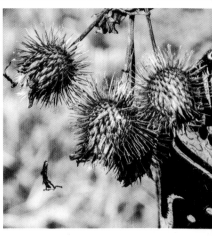

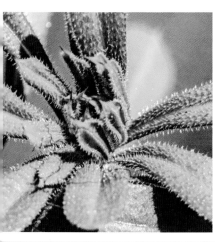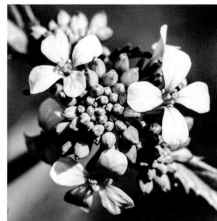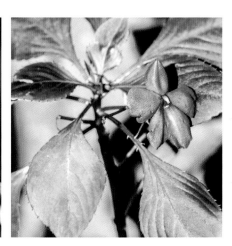

WEEDS

Understanding Nature's Little Workers

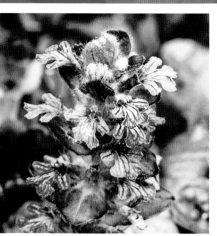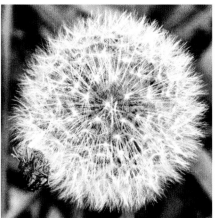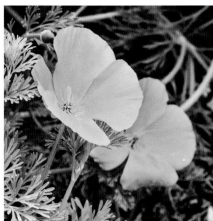

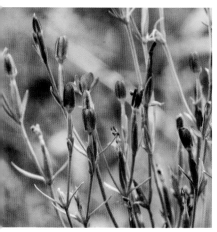

Pat Collins

Photography by Glen Collins

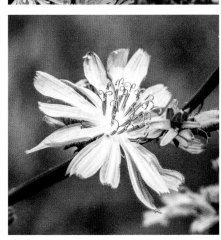

First published in 2017 by New Holland Publishers Pty Ltd
London • Sydney • Auckland

The Chandlery, Unit 704, 50 Westminster Bridge Road, London SE1 7QY, UK
1/66 Gibbes Street, Chatswood, NSW 2067, Australia
5/39 Woodside Avenue, Northcote, Auckland 0627, New Zealand

www.newhollandpublishers.com

Copyright © 2017 New Holland Publishers Pty Ltd
Copyright © 2017 in text: Pat Collins
Copyright © 2017 in images: Glen Collins,
    except Mullein and Hawthorn, which were supplied by Laura Skykes.

All rights reserved. No part of this publication may be reproduced, stored in a retrieval system or transmitted, in any form or by any means, electronic, mechanical, photocopying, recording or otherwise, without the prior written permission of the publishers and copyright holders.

A record of this book is held at the British Library and the National Library of Australia.

ISBN 9781921517792

Group Managing Director: Fiona Schultz
Publisher: Diane Ward
Project Editor: Liz Hardy
Designer: Andrew Davies
Production Director: James Mills-Hicks
Printer: Times International Printers, Malaysia

10 9 8 7 6 5 4 3 2 1

Keep up with New Holland Publishers on Facebook
www.facebook.com/NewHollandPublishers

Dedication

To Mum.
Thank you for being such a wonderful positive influence on my life.

Acknowledgements

I would like to thank my son Glen who is responsible for all the high quality pictures in this book except for Mullein and Hawthorn which, were supplied by Laura Sykes. I would also like to thank the dedication of Ross-Lyn, one of my receptionists, for all the work she did to complete the book. Other helpers and proofreaders are my mother, Robert and Denise – thank you so much for your time. My daughter Kim also helped with reference material. There have been many other helpers along my path who I would also like to thank, especially my husband Bryant for putting up with all the long hours I spent on the book. Last but not least a big thankyou to Buddhi who encouraged me to write this book and found my publishers New Holland Publishers.

In touch with the earth

Hi, I'm Pat Collins, welcome to my wondrous world of weeds. What made you pick up this book? Are you inquisitive and just want to know what those pesky weeds are and if they have any uses; are you a farmer or hobby farmer and want to know what weeds indicate about your soil and how you can use them on the farm or are you just interested in living more sustainably with nature? This book will help you with all these questions.

What made me so interested in weeds? I need to go back to my childhood, which was spent on dairy farms in the Hunter Valley of NSW, north of Sydney. I knew about Catheads, as they got stuck in my feet, and Saffron Thistle, as it would hurt my bare legs. I remember Bathurst Burr, which attached itself to the cows' tails and Mallow that covered the yards. However, my favorite was Stinking Roger, as I loved crushing and smelling it. The memories and smells of the weeds from your childhood stay with you.

I grew up, left the farm life and moved into town, working as a clerical assistant, but my love of plants stayed with me. I used to have a pet goat that I would lead down to the river to feed and would watch all the different plants she would graze on. My future husband Bryant and I bought a hard, dry patch of land near Muswellbrook, and took out our goat, and we soon had quite a menagerie.

My son Glen was born out on this property before we moved to a patch of nearby wilderness we still call home at Martindale, surrounded by Wollemi National Park. We had poor access and no power but it was green with a creek and 100 hectares (247 acres) of land for our stock. I have always been into self-sufficiency and we built our house, milked our goats and cow, got honey from our bees, grew our vegetables and fruit and so much more. My daughter Kim was soon born to complete our little family.

When my youngest was only two years old I became interested in studying herbs by correspondence. This opened a new world for me. This course taught me I could use herbs to help with health issues and a large number of those herbs were weeds that grew at my doorstep. I was hooked! The more I learnt, the more I wanted to learn. Wow, I could use Chickweed and Plantain for eczema and Nettles for my hair. This was unreal! I started to experiment and made my own ointments, creams and syrups. My children were my guinea pigs and put up with me trialing poultices, syrups and oils.

I completed a Diploma in Herbal Medicine in 1989 and then went on to do other courses. Around this time a friend asked me if I wanted to teach gardening at our local TAFE college. I agreed, and my first course was in the town that I was born in – Denman. My students were keen and I decided to teach them about how to use the weeds that grew in their backyard. We did a six-month course and covered every common illness: making an ointment for skin problems, a soothing cream, cough syrups, teas and so much more. This course proved to be popular and for the next twenty years I taught all around the district and beyond. I taught thousands of people and they in turn taught their families and friends. My students proudly talked about their medicine chests full of potions they had made with me. They used them on unsuspecting visitors with great results.

After a request from TAFE and having heard all my students' stories I started to write my books. I called them *In Touch with the Earth* as I felt people were starting to lose touch with Mother Earth. The first book was *A–Z of Ailments* followed by *Oh No Not the Onion Poultice Again*, which was full of stories of how I used my remedies on my family. Then came my first recipe book, *Pat's Herbal Recipes* followed by *Useful Weeds at our Doorstep*. These last two books have been my biggest sellers. Later on I wrote a book on herbs in the home garden called *Medicinal Herbs for Home Use*, a book on bush tucker and survival, *Bush Wise* and *More Recipes from Pat*. I also had a DVD made that I based on my *A–Z of Ailments*. My first book was written in 1995 and last one 2007. In between, many things had happened.

In 1994, I decided with much persuasion by my students to start practicing as a herbalist. I started working a few days a week at a teahouse and in 1997 moved on to buy the building we now call Total Health and Education Centre (THE Centre). A few fellow practitioners helped me start and it has gone from strength to strength. Now I sell a large range of my products at THE Centre and four days a week I run my busy practice as a herbalist.

At the same time, I kept doing something I love, and that was teaching. I now only teach private workshops and courses, often traveling long distances to do so. In addition, I am employed to teach Manufacturing and Botany at a college in the city of Newcastle. I am teaching our future naturopaths and herbalists and take pride in doing that job. I am often asked to be a guest speaker and volunteer my time for any community group. I love passing on my knowledge.

My husband and I still live on our property at Martindale surrounded by the peace and tranquility of hills covered in native flora. We have so many different birds and other wildlife and I have an old dog, my mate Boxer, 12 chooks and numerous cattle that have decided to take off over the hills due to recent fires clearing the scrub. I am surrounded by my gardens, fruit trees and other trees and bushes. My garden is also home for numerous weeds that I eat on a regular basis and use in my herbal preparations. I enjoy their variety and their ability to attract insects such as butterflies and bees.

This gives you my background and some understanding as to why I have written this book. I also love to share my knowledge and I want you to understand how you can live with nature by understanding her little workers.

What is a weed?

What is the meaning of a weed? The Macquarie Dictionary states that it is 'a plant growing wild, especially in cultivated ground to the exclusion or injury of the desired crop.' Weeds are referred to as a plant out of place. If White Clover covers your lawn and the flowers attract bees, you worry about treading on them so class this plant as a weed. If Chickweed is growing all over your vegetable garden and smothering it or Mallow is taking over a patch of your garden these would also be called weeds. Once you understand the uses of weeds, you could look at these three plants differently: Clover is improving your ground with nitrogen and you can eat the flowers; Chickweed is a delicious salad green and the chooks adore it and Mallows are reconditioning your soil and it makes a great ointment.

The students I teach love learning about using the weeds instead of killing them. I always remember John, an elderly gentleman on one of my Denman courses who told me he used a Weed Wand to get rid of all those pesky Dandelions ruining his lovely green lawn. After being at my course for six months he came back to do the course again. This time he came laden with a box of Dandelion leaves he had picked for the students to use. Wonderful students like John have taught me so much. We are often ignorant of what grows around us. We know our vegetables and fruit trees, a good lawn grass and some pretty flowers but know little about those troublesome plants that grow in our gardens destroying our pretty straight lines and competing for room with what we have planted.

I do not just teach students I also teach my clients about how to use plants if they are interested. One lovely lady had many health problems including deafness, several forms of arthritis and cancer. She wanted what she called natural 'chemotherapy'. She just wanted to grow plants that she could use to maintain her health. I told her about Plantain and Clivers. Immediately she planted a row of Plantain on either side of her path and got her father to collect the Clivers that grew in paddocks nearby. She uses these plants in her daily juice and over the last ten years she has been able to maintain her health. Those rows of Plantain on either side of her path are a picture with their tall seed heads and long, ribbed leaves.

I could tell you so many stories of people who now use weeds in their life whereas once they would have trodden on them or dug them up. It is just knowledge and that is what I want to impart to you.

This book is a culmination of my life's work on understanding and using weeds. They are part of my life. Just this morning I picked some fresh lettuce leaves, along with other plants coming up in my vegie patch. I picked tender Chickweed, Sow Thistle, Dandelion,

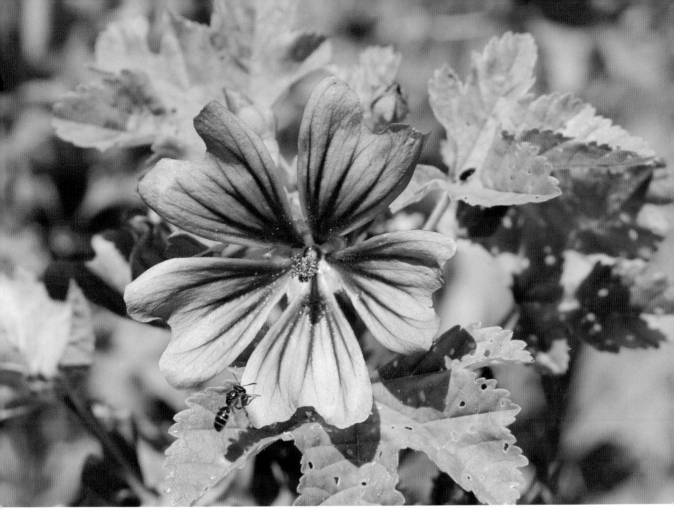

Fat Hen and Amaranth leaves but decided to refrain from picking the Nettles. On the weekend, I had picked a basket full of Nettles and put them in my drying shed. This weekend I will be picking the tops of the Stinking Roger plant and putting them into olive oil to create an insect-repellent oil.

When I was researching this book, I found uses for numerous plants I didn't know about. I can't tell you how excited I was when I found there was a use for my pesky Farmer's Friends. Finding out how much research there is on Nut Grass was also a great find. Then I had to sample all my wild Brassicas trying to work out which one was which. Hedge mustard, also known as Singer's Plant, and used for sore throats is definitely something I will be trialing soon. Wait until you read about Prickly Pear and how it is used for diabetes and what great potential weeds like Jerusalem Artichokes have for biomass.

We now have information readily available. Just ask a question and I am sure Google has the answer. In fact, we have information overload and how do we tell fact from a belief? When I was writing this book I decided I would have to do a lot of research to back up my own and traditional knowledge. Thanks to sites like Google Scholar and looking up published medical research papers (Pubmed) we have information from all over the world. It is amazing how much research there is on our weeds and the citations are impressive.

When I first started writing this book I had a few ideas in mind. Firstly, I wanted to write a book I wish someone had written 30 years ago when I started on this pathway. I wanted a book with clear and accurate photos to help with identification (often why people avoid trialing a weed). To back this up, a simple description was important along with information on where it came from and if it grew in my area. Then, instead of the usual weed books you find that tell you how to poison it, I wanted to list its uses. Is it edible or medicinal and can I use it for other purposes like dyes and perfumes? I felt it was important to explain its impact on the farm: will this weed poison my stock, can I make use of this weed and what does it do to the environment? Coming from a farming background myself, I know farmers want to know how to manage their weeds and many want to get away from herbicides. This information is also useful on a smaller scale in the home garden. Lastly, I decided to write about why the weed grew where it did (e.g. soil high in iron or impacted).

Weeds fall into many categories. Some of the most prolific weeds have followed man such as Plantain, Dandelions, Fat Hen and Sow Thistle. Others grown for their beauty or medicinal value have escaped cultivation such as many of our flowers like Nasturtium, Sweet Briar, Agapanthus and Elder. Trees once popular such as Peppercorn and Honey Locust are now reclassified as weeds. Many humans have grown plants for a specific reason such as Hawthorn as a hedge, Prickly Pear for the fruits and Water Hyacinth to beautify our waterways. Numerous weeds are spread by animals, birds and pollen blown by the wind, some over great distances.

I sometimes think humans are like weeds. We usually come from another country and populate a new niche wiping out flora and fauna as we spread our civilization. Doesn't that sound like our invasive weeds that we poison to keep in control?!

I am aware that weeds are one of the major factors affecting Australia's biodiversity and agriculture. Weeds, like humans, change the functioning of natural ecosystems. Read about Spiny Emex that has taken over native flora and so the birds have adapted and now eat its fruit instead. All I am asking is that we look outside the square and realize why the weed has become rampant. It may be due to mineral imbalances in the soil. Often minerals that are high in the soil are locked in by another minderal imbalance and weeds will try to uptake them. That is why they make good green crops and compost. If you wish to get rid of an infestation then cut them down, add the minerals that are low, drain the land, add humus or compost and aerate the impacted soils. This is so much better than our modern day use of herbicides, which often create a hardpan and make the land unproductive.

Nature is constantly trying to fix our mistakes. It grows plants that will balance the soil. With their deep taproots, Mallow and Dandelion will open up the soil, bring minerals to the surface then break down to humus. It may take years for nature to correct man's mistakes, but she is patient. We need to be more in tune with her needs and watch and understand how she works.

Another important thing about this book is that it helps with self-reliance; a better word than self-sufficiency. Only 200 years ago we were mostly slaves or serfs to a master. Now in today's civilized world we are slaves to media and the world of consumerism. Most of us don't even know where our food comes from. So few people grow their own and our farmers make up a minute part of our population. We need to take back control and learn about the plants around us. A plant might help stop your diarrhea or cold, be a survival food, and another might be used to thatch a roof for shelter. This is important in today's changing world where we feel unsure of the future.

I started writing a simple book but it soon grew as I covered all the aspects of weeds. I tried to include a wide variety of weeds, some you will recognize growing in your garden, often as a flower, others as pesky plants in the garden or paddock and yet others majestic trees. The majority of these weeds grow worldwide so are easy to find wherever you go. Weeds follow mankind and after you have read this book you will realize they will also help us with your health and wellbeing. Just stop a moment, smell the air, watch the birds and the butterflies and see the flowers open their petals to the sun. Let us be at peace with the earth, stop trying to dominate it, work with it instead. Look at those weeds you once thought of as a nuisance and understand how they fix the earth, putting nutrients back into the soil so that we can grow produce high in nutrients. If you look after Mother Nature, she will in turn look after you. On the other hand, if you want to fight her by using poisons she will bide her time then patiently try to fix up our mistakes. Be gentle with the Earth as she is all we have and presently we are reaping the damage we are doing. Our poisons are causing imbalance to the ecosystem and our food is lacking nutrients due to impacted soils with locked and imbalanced minerals. Only you can make a difference and I hope this book will help you follow a new path of understanding.

There are many people I must thank that have helped me make this book and they will be in the acknowledgements. However, I must thank my son Glen most of all as without him I doubt if there would be a book. He has taken some outstanding photos and enhanced mine as well to create a fantastic tool for identification. He has been tireless in helping create this book on the computer, which has been a bit of a nightmare! I am no computer guru, I learn as I go and you should have seen the mess I made of recording the research. We've had lots of long days and nights finishing this book and I do hope you will enjoy it as much as we did creating it. Keep in touch and share your stories.

Pat Collins 2016

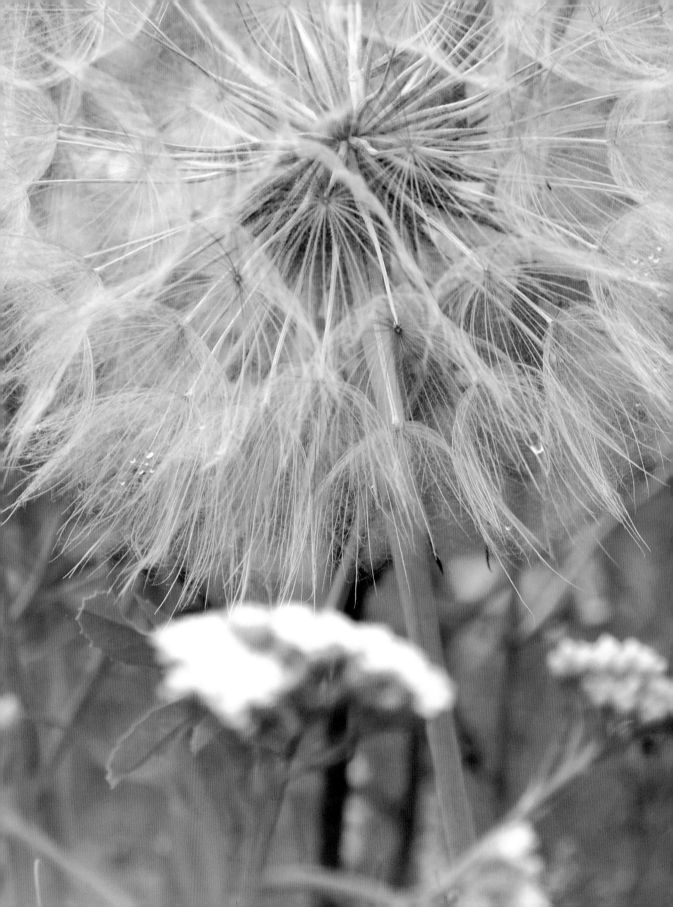

The Weeds

AGAPANTHUS

African lily

Agapanthus praecox subs. *orientalis*

DISTRIBUTION Native to South Africa and now widespread. Naturalized in southern Australia, mainly Tasmania.

HABITAT Grown as an ornamental that has escaped. Growing in gardens, roadsides, edge of forests, wastelands and disturbed sites.

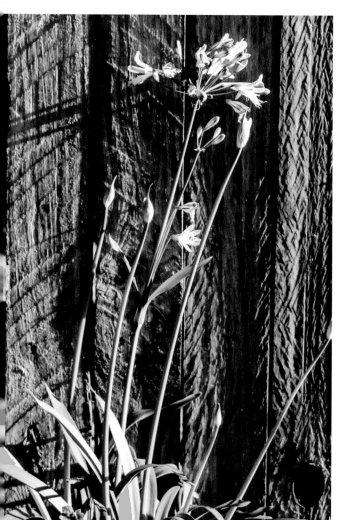

DESCRIPTION

Perennial plant with a flowering stalk up to 120 cm (3 ft 9 in) tall. Strong underground rhizome system.

LEAVES Large, leathery, strap-like, which grow in clusters from the base of the plant.

FLOWERS Generally blue with six large petals that are fused into a tube at the base.

FRUIT/SEED Large, elongated, three-sided capsule full of seeds.

USES

EDIBLE/OTHER Considered a magical and medicinal plant by the indigenous people of South Africa. Tins and old pots of Agapanthus are grown around the home as they are considered a plant of fertility and pregnancy. To

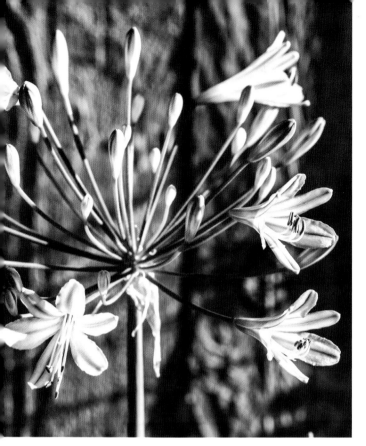
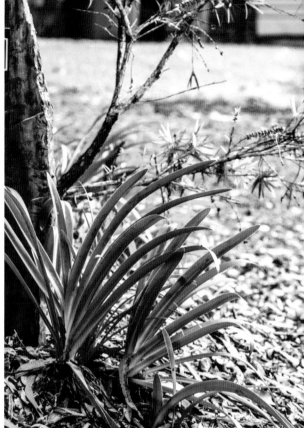

soothe your feet after a long hike, weave the soft leaves into a slipper shape, put over the feet and relax. Has a silky smoothness that eases your aches. Use the leaf as a bandage to hold a poultice.[1]

MEDICINAL Xhosa women of South Africa use the root for pregnancy and childbirth. Zulu use the plant for heart disease, paralysis, an emetic for coughs, colds, chest pains and tightness.[1] This plant contains toxins and I wonder if these locals have built up a resistance to the toxins. Advised not to take internally. Externally the juice from the rhizome is antifungal.

FARM/ENVIR. When I was in southern Queensland, I noticed that Agapanthus grew on the edge of the forests, multiplying via their rhizomes. It is such an easy plant to grow and you are rewarded with a long period of flowering. Agapanthus come in many varieties and colors and people make good money from selling the flower heads, especially the white ones for weddings. Stock seem to avoid eating the plant as the leaves have an acrid sap. Dig it out of your paddocks as it contains toxins.

FURTHER READING *Indigenous Healing Plants* by Margaret Roberts (AGAPANTHUS).[1]

WARNING Toxic to humans and the sticky acrid sap in the leaves can cause severe ulceration of the mouth. May be a skin irritant.

AMARANTH

Redroot and Green Amaranth

Amaranthus retroflexus, Amaranthus viridis

DISTRIBUTION Redroot Amaranth originated from North America and now grows worldwide. Naturalized in southern and eastern Australia. Green Amaranth is cosmopolitan and found in tropical, subtropical and temperate regions of the world. Naturalized throughout Australia.

HABITAT Both Amaranths are vigorous weeds of summer crops and found in wastelands, disturbed areas, gardens and horticulture.

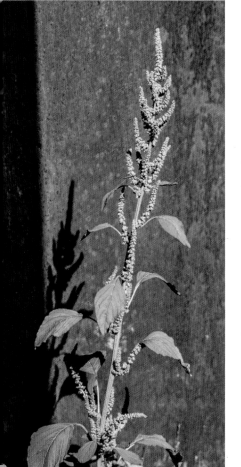

DESCRIPTION

Both are shrubby annual erect weeds growing to 1 m (3 ft 3 in) in height and branches may get a reddish tinge. Redroot Amaranth can grow taller, its stems have dense hairs and its taproot is pinkish to red.

LEAVES Both Amaranths have alternate green leaves with prominent veins on long stalks, oval to lance-like. Redroot Amaranth leaves are coarser than Green Amaranth.

FLOWERS Redroot Amaranth has a bristly seed spike that has small inconspicuous flowers that grow terminally and in upper leaf axils. Green Amaranth has small green flowers sometimes with a reddish tinge also growing in dense spikes, often many branched.

FRUIT/SEED Redroot Amaranth has glossy, round, small black seeds, which are released from tiny capsules. Green Amaranth has wrinkled fruit capsules, which are small, brown, and do not open to release the seeds when ripe. The seeds are tiny, smooth and glossy.

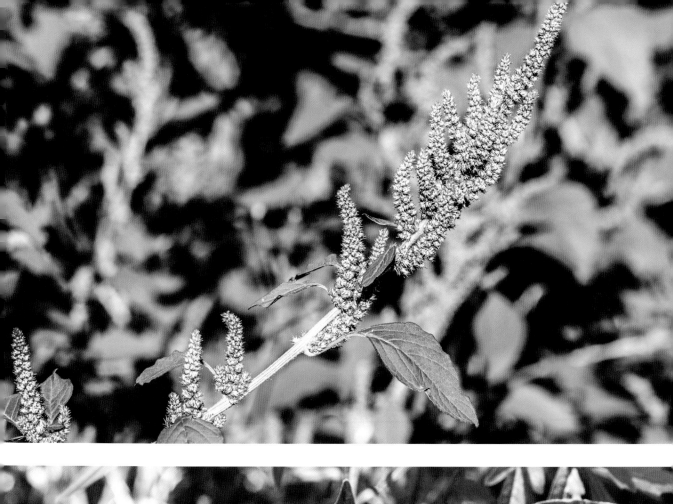
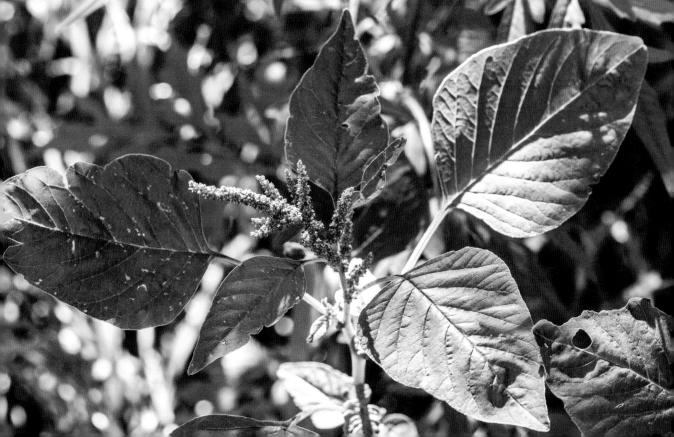

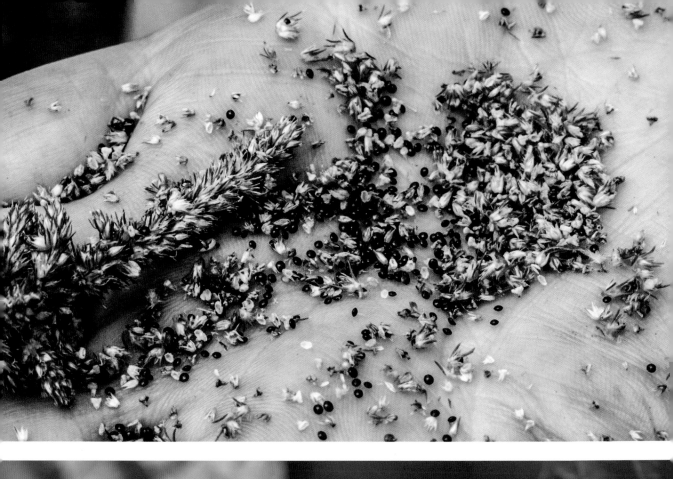
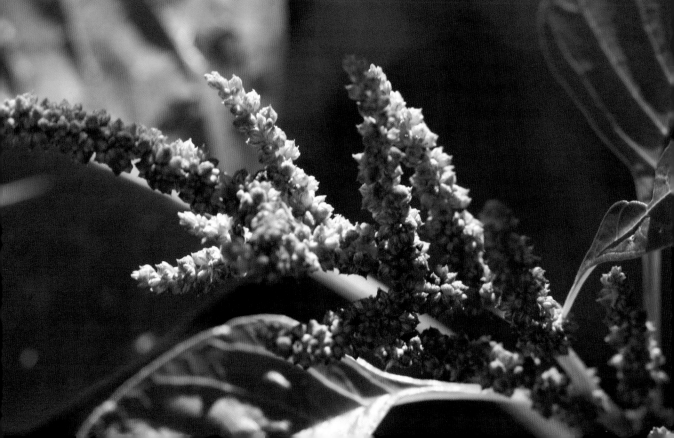

USES

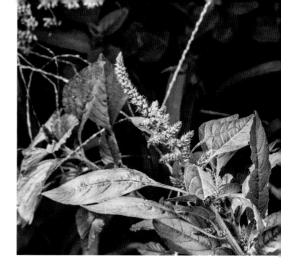

EDIBLE/OTHER There are a handful of edible species of Amaranth that have been cultivated for their grain for thousands of years. Of the many weed species, *Amaranthus hybridus* is the only worthwhile weedy species to grow as a crop. However, Green Amaranth makes an excellent pot herb used like spinach, containing large amounts of protein, vitamins and minerals. The seeds, although small and hard to grind are also nutritious and used in a wide variety of dishes. Redroot Amaranth leaves are also a spinach substitute but I find them coarser, higher in oxalate content and with very little flavor and I prefer the Green Amaranth's leaves. They are high in iron and vitamin A. After winnowing, the seeds are roasted to improve flavor and are easier to grind. Add to your baking. I do enjoy these seeds but beware it takes many hours to fill a small jar. This amaranth also makes green and yellow dye.

MEDICINAL Redroot Amaranth leaves are astringent and made into a tea for diarrhea, dysentery and gastro disorders and the plant juice is taken for excessive menstruation. Used externally to treat inflammations and internally for fluid problems. Also used for throat and mouth infections. Green Amaranth is popular in Ayurvedic medicine as a tonic, for kidney ailments, dysentery, worming, as a cough remedy and is even used for convulsions. Externally, poultices are used to treat inflammation, boils, abscesses and hemorrhoids.

FARM/ENVIR. Redroot Amaranth is an aggressive and competitive weed in a variety of crops and has allelopathic effects on both weeds and crops. It is an alternative host for a number of crop pests and diseases. Green Amaranth is very common and can be a serious weed in virtually any crop. It usually grows with other weeds. Both species are high in nutrients and make excellent fodder and green manure crops. Best in mixed pasture. Indicates soil low in calcium and phosphate and very high in potassium and magnesium, low in humus and bacteria, with good drainage and a hard crust. [8]

MAY BE CONFUSED WITH Many other species of Amaranths and most are edible, however, note the dense, hairy stems and spikes of Redroot Amaranth and the wrinkled seeds of Green Amaranth.

FURTHER READING *Amaranthus viridis*, reduced elevated blood glucose level, improved lipid profile in induced diabetic rats.[2]

WARNING Under certain conditions, nitrates and oxalates may reach toxic levels (Redroot Amaranth). Amaranths can cause allergic reactions in humans due to wind-borne pollen.

ANGLED ONION

Onion Weed, Three-cornered Leek, Three-cornered Garlic

Allium triquetrum

DISTRIBUTION Native to the Mediterranean region and now worldwide. Naturalized in southern Australia.

HABITAT Found in gardens, wastelands, waterways, dairy grazing areas, orchards and along roadsides.

DESCRIPTION

A clumping plant growing 30–50 cm (12–20 in) tall.

LEAVES Green and grass-like, appearing after the autumn rains and dying down in winter.

FLOWERS The charming, white, bell flowers grow on long stalks and have a pale green stripe in the center of each petal. They flower in clusters of about five flowers and nod towards the ground in spring and summer.

FRUIT/SEED Numerous oblong black seeds.

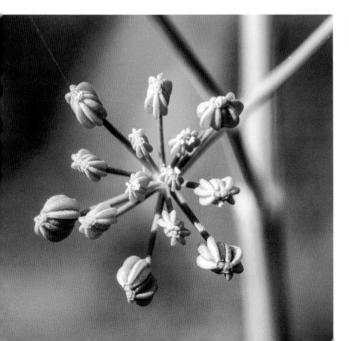
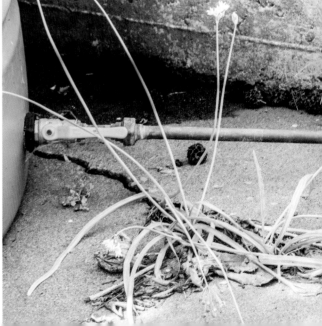

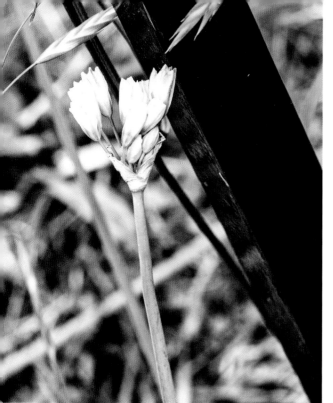
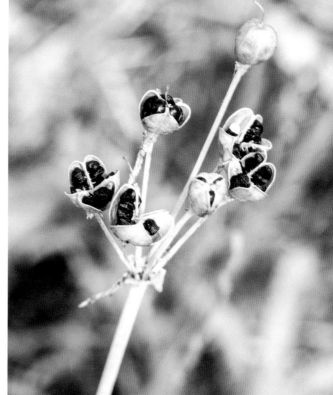

USES

EDIBLE/OTHER Eat bulbs, flowers and stems. This plant is in the onion family and has a slightly onion/garlic flavor. A good spring onion (scallion) substitute. It contains sulfur, which gives it its characteristic smell. Best eaten raw in salads to retain its delicate flavor. May be cooked like leeks but will lose flavor and become fibrous. Use the bulbs when the plant dies down. Also known as an insect repellent.

MEDICINAL Containing sulfur, which is an important mineral in a healthy diet.

FARM/ENVIR. Noxious weed in the southern states of Australia. It taints milk and meat even in low densities. May grow in large clumps and can be difficult to remove as any little bulb left in the ground will germinate. Mowing low to the ground, grazing cattle and eating the bulbs are all good strategies to clear up infested areas. I found it popping up in my garden in town and was pleased to find it has uses.

MAY BE CONFUSED WITH Cultivated Snowdrops (*Leucojum vernum*) which have no smell and a green spot on petals.

FURTHER READING Saponins and flavonoids of *Allium triquetrum*.[3]

WARNING Contact dermatitis for people with sensitive skin. Organosulfur compounds that are in the onion and garlic families may be potentially toxic to susceptible dogs and cats.

BATHURST BURR

Thorny Cocklebur

Xanthium spinosum

DISTRIBUTION Native of South America, now a widespread weed naturalized in Australia and throughout the world except for tropical regions.

HABITAT Classified as one of the world's worst weeds it is highly invasive growing in summer crops, abundant in pastures, cultivation and wasteland.

DESCRIPTION

A coarse annual herb which may become woody and bushy. Stems have many groups of three-pronged, stiff, yellowish spines at the base of each leaf or branch.

LEAVES Dark green with prominent white veins, lighter underneath due to covering of fine hairs. Leaves divided into three irregular lobes.

FLOWERS Male flowers are numerous, tiny flowers arranged in clusters on tips of stems, yellow to creamy-white in color. Female flowers are greenish colored, borne singly or in small clusters in upper leaf forks. Fruiting in warmer months.

FRUIT/SEED Fruit is greenish when young then straw colored and brown when mature. Oval shaped burr covered in numerous small, hooked spines with two small spines at the tip, which contains two seeds.

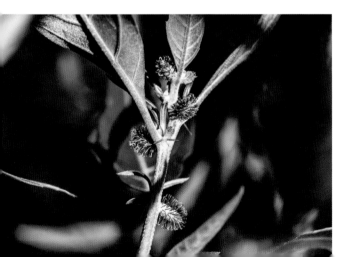
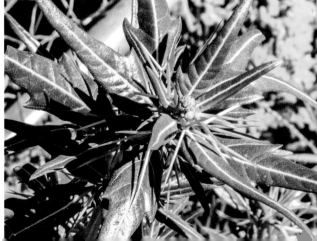

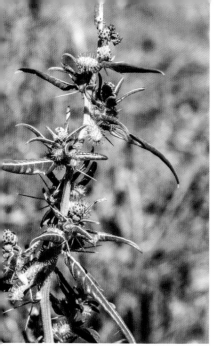
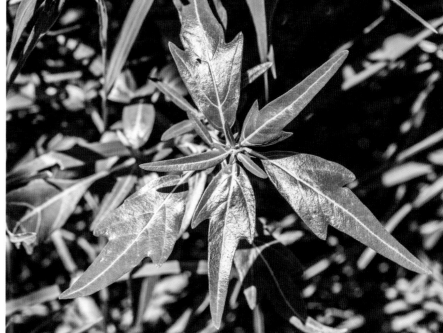

USES

EDIBLE/OTHER This plant is not edible. Produces a yellow dye.

MEDICINAL In Argentina, the leaves are used for backache and for cleansing the blood. In Europe, the leaves used as an infusion for the treatment of hydrophobia, for fevers and to stop bleeding. In addition, an extract of the roots is taken for digestive problems.

FARM/ENVIR. An economically serious weed in Australia and in many other countries. Declared noxious in the state of New South Wales. Spread by burrs clinging to animal fur, clothing etc. and dispersed in weedy hay and impure seed stocks. I remember in my childhood on the dairy farm the cow's tails covered in these burrs lashing our poor faces when milking. Poisoning has occurred in pigs and other animals when they have eaten the young, palatable plants. (A large pig would have to ingest 500 seedlings to be poisoned.) Animals will avoid grazing on older plants. I have found hoeing every summer after the rains, when they appear, will keep the numbers manageable.

MAY BE CONFUSED WITH Other plants in the Xanthium genus. The four species that grow in Australia are Hunter Burr (*X. italicum*), South American Burr (*X. cavanillesii*), Californian Burr (*X. orientale*) and Noogoora Burr (*X. occidentale*). All with maple-like leaves and their own variations. See *Weeds, An illustrated botanical guide*.

FURTHER READING Xanthatin and xanthinosin from burrs as potential anticancer agent.[4] Antiarthritic activity of *Xanthium strumarium* L.[5]

WARNING Young seedlings contain sulfated glycosides, which are toxic. Toxicity decreases, as they get older.

BILLYGOAT WEED

Common Billygoat Weed, Blue Billygoat Weed

Ageratum conyzoides, Ageratum houstonianum

DISTRIBUTION Originated from tropical Central and South America. Now naturalized in subtropical and tropical countries of the world. Found in the wetter parts of Australia, especially the eastern coastal districts.

HABITAT Garden escapee now in disturbed sites, roadsides, waste areas, along watercourses, forests, grasslands and cultivated areas.

DESCRIPTION

Both are weakly erect, short-lived annuals, slightly aromatic with shallow roots identified by their fluffy, flowering clusters.

LEAVES Pale green, softly hairy and opposite.

FLOWERS Common Billygoat are white, blue or mauve and the back of the bracts around the flower heads are sparsely hairy or hairless. Blue Billygoat are blue-mauve to pink-mauve and the back of their bracts are densely hairy. Flowers throughout the year.

FRUIT/SEED Small, brown, one-seeded.

USES

EDIBLE/OTHER These plants are not edible.

MEDICINAL In both species the juice is used externally for treating burns and wounds and both have insecticidal activity. Common Billygoat is used more extensively in traditional medicine, especially in Brazil where the whole plant is made into a tea and taken for colic, colds, fevers, diarrhea, rheumatism, spasms, burns and wounds. Other uses are to treat headache, pneumonia and as an antibacterial agent. I collect my plants for medicinal use from areas where the plant has naturalized and in this case I collect them in the subtropical area of Mapleton, Queensland where my mother lives.

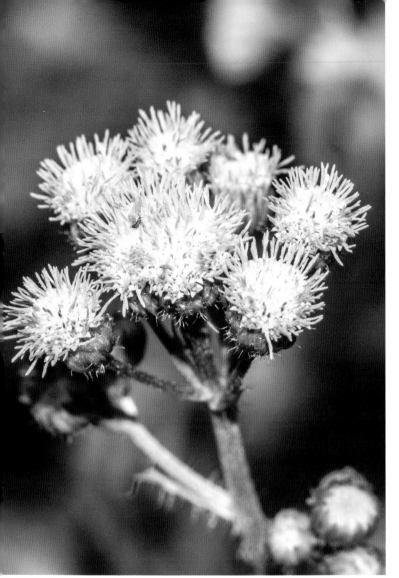
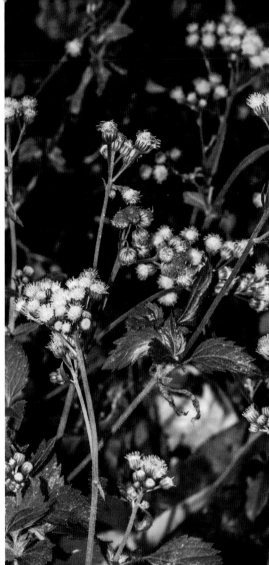

FARM/ENVIR. Important weed in all crops in tropics and subtropics as first species to colonize degraded areas and prevent other plants establishing. Has allelopathic properties that inhibits the growth and germination of other plants. Forms dense stands and is prone to being a rampant environmental weed. Has a life cycle of only two months and easily pulled out of the ground if you have a small infestation. Shown in research to be effective against mosquitoes, cattle ticks and other insects.[6a]

FURTHER READING Pharmacological investigations and insecticidal activities outlined in many research papers. Effect of *Ageratum houstonianum* Mill. (Asteraceae) leaf extracts on the oviposition activity.[6] In vitro evaluation of ethanolic extracts of *Ageratum conyzoides*.[6a] *Ageratum conyzoides* L. (Asteraceae).[7]

BISHOP'S WEED

False Queen Anne's Lace, Bishop's Flower

Ammi majus

DISTRIBUTION Native to North Africa, Europe and Asia now widespread in temperate zones. In Australia, grows throughout New South Wales, south-east Queensland and in Victoria.

HABITAT Grown as an ornamental and now a garden escapee growing in crops, pastures, disturbed sites and natural habitats.

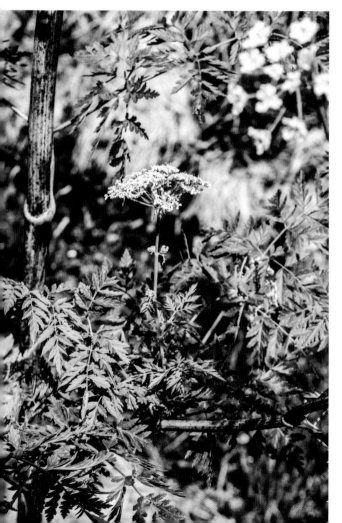

DESCRIPTION

Erect, annual, hairless herb.

LEAF Lower leaves divided and the upper ones finely dissected.

FLOWER In the Umbelliferae family so the flowers look like umbrellas of small white flowers on top of stalks.

FRUIT/SEED Two oblong segments with ridges containing seeds.

USES

EDIBLE/OTHER Seed used as a condiment. Medicinal seeds used as a contraceptive, for fluid problems, kidney stones, urinary infections, asthma, menstruation, angina and as a tonic. Also antibacterial, antifungicidal and used to treat psoriasis and vitiligo.

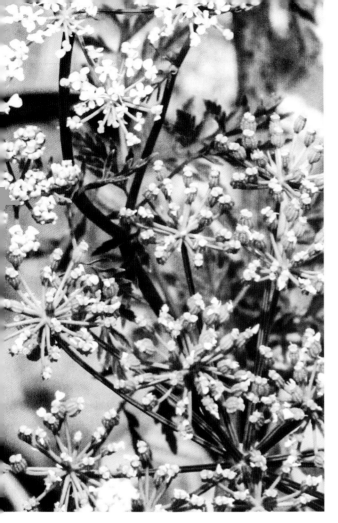
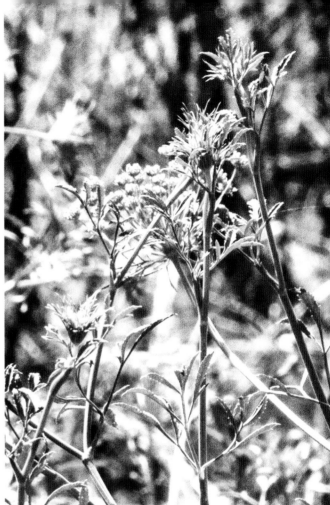

FARM/ENVIR. Still grown in cottage style gardens. Pest in crops, especially cotton, and has become a bad environmental weed, especially in New South Wales and Victoria. Threatening many conservation sites and significant natural habitats. Moderately palatable with stock and low risk to goats. Avoid grazing animals in infested areas when the plant seeds.

MAY BE CONFUSED WITH This plant closely resembles the deadly Hemlock (*Conium maculatum*) but it does not have its distinct mousy odor or purple spots on the stems and leaf stalks. Wild Carrot or Queen Anne's Lace (*Daucus carota*), which is similar but the root has a distinct carrot odor.

FURTHER READING Effect of *Trigonella foenum-graecum* and *Ammi majus* on calcium oxalate urolithiasis in rats.[14]

WARNING Some sensitive people develop skin problems when touching the plant and the fruit may cause hayfever. Seeds contains furanocoumarins, which are toxic to stock. Nitrate poisoning may also occur but animals are not affected if they eat small amounts.

BLACK THISTLE

Bull Thistle

Cirsium vulgare

DISTRIBUTION Native to Europe, western Asia and North Africa and now flourishing throughout the temperate zones of the world. Found in all states of Australia except the Northern Territory.

HABITAT Like all thistles, it flourishes in highly fertile soils growing in pastures, old cultivation wasteland and roadsides.

DESCRIPTION

Annual or biennial erect hairy plant up to 150 cm (4 ft 9 in) tall with furrowed and winged stems branching in upper parts.

LEAVES Dark green above, white woolly beneath with each lobe ending in a sharp rigid spine.

FLOWERS Globular, purple head surrounded by spiny bracts. Flowers summer/autumn.

FRUIT/SEED Small light colored, topped with a downy pappus.

USES

EDIBLE/OTHER This is a renowned survival food. You can cook the roots, although they taste bland and can cause gas. Leaves can be eaten once the spines are taken off but I've found there isn't much left to eat! The stems before flowering, with the spiky rind taken off, can be eaten raw or cooked and taste like chokos. Purple heads used as chewing gum or chewing tobacco by American Indians. Dried flowers can be used as a rennet substitute to curdle milk. Other uses are the seed's oil content, the downy fiber makes excellent tinder and paper can be made from the fiber of the stems.

MEDICINAL To relieve piles take herb internally and apply a poultice if needed. Use

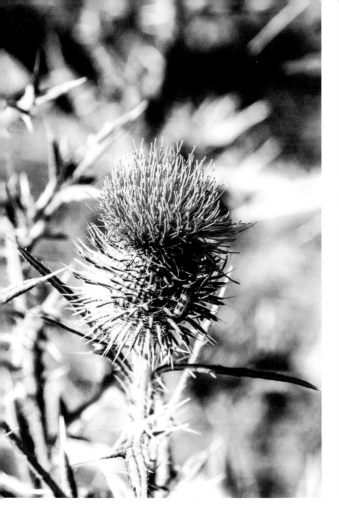
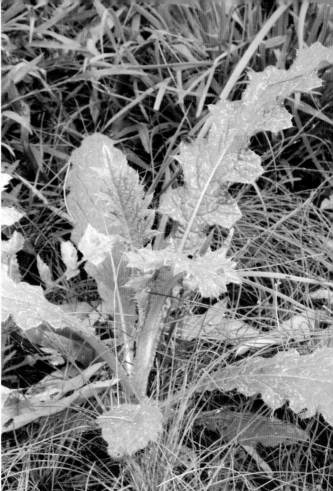

internally for rheumatic conditions, joint pains, stomach cramps, inflammation and for antibacterial and antifungal problems.

FARM/ENVIR. Most widespread thistle in Australia and a nuisance in agriculture and pastures. This thistle grows all over our top paddock but because it is not a heavy infestation, it is manageable. I also find the deep roots bring up nutrients and the grasses around its base thrive. Thistle leaves, crushed in a mill to destroy prickles, make good cattle fodder. Its presence indicates soil low in calcium, but high in magnesium, iron and other minerals, low in humus with compacted soils.[8]

MAY BE CONFUSED WITH Scotch Thistle (*Onopordum acanthium*) as the heads are similar however the plant is whitish-grey with woolly stems and leaves. Also not as common or widespread as Black Thistle.

FURTHER READING Evaluation of putative cytotoxic activity of crude extracts from *Onopordum acanthium* leaves – antitumor and immune related activity.[9]

BLACKBERRY

Bramble

Rubus fruticosus

DISTRIBUTION Native to Europe and now worldwide. Found in all states of Australia.

HABITAT Serious and noxious weed of forests, creeks, riverbanks, roadsides and pastures enjoying cooler, high-rainfall areas.

DESCRIPTION

Erect woody shrub up to 5 m (16 ft) high with scrambling, prickly stems up to 6 m (20 ft) long. Stems may root at tips.

LEAVES Three to five evenly or irregularly toothed leaflets, white underneath with prickly leaf stalks.

FLOWERS White to pink, five petals in clusters at end of branches.

FRUIT/SEED Berries are globular in shape made up of an aggregate of one-seeded fruits, which ripen from green to red to black in summer. Seeds are light to dark brown, deeply and irregularly pitted.

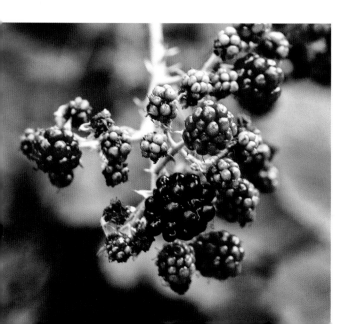

USES

EDIBLE/OTHER Fruits eaten since Neolithic times and used for wines, syrups, jams, jellies, pies, teas, vinegars and soups. High in vitamin C, iron and antioxidants. To collect you should ensure you have boots, tough jeans and long sleeve shirt as the lethal thorns hook into bare skin and clothes. I carry many a scar from bushes growing in the National Park

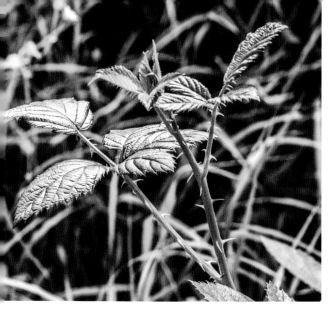
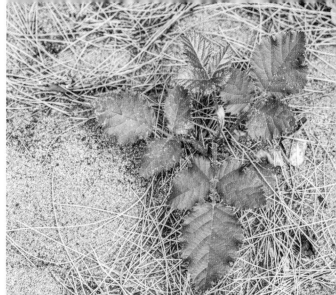

nearby. In a good season well worth picking. Be careful if picking in an area you don't know as Blackberries are a noxious weed and often sprayed with strong herbicides. You can also enjoy a spring salad of Blackberry shoots. Pick before they develop prickles, peel and chop them and add to your favorite salad.

MEDICINAL Useful in the treatment of cancer, dysentery, diarrhea, whooping cough, colitis, toothache, anemia, psoriasis, sore throat, mouth ulcer, mouthwash, hemorrhoids, and minor bleeding. Also used as an antimicrobial, antioxidant, for dysentery and diabetes.[10a] Fruits are made into syrups and juices, leaves into tea and roots ground, dried and used as a decoction.

FARM/ENVIR. Millions are spent in Australia trying to eradicate this weed. In Europe, grown as part of the fenceline creating a thick, impenetrable natural barrier. Often home for rabbits and foxes. Goats will eat the tips and keep the plants in check but avoid using mohair goats — they get really tangled! Cows with bloat and calves with worms will right themselves on a diet of Blackberry leaves. Spanish gypsies gave their horses an infusion of Blackberry leaves if they needed a tonic. A poultice from crushed Blackberry roots is used to treat eczema and other skin diseases in animals. Worldwide there are 2,000 named species and subspecies of *R. fruticosus*. Indicates soil low in calcium and phosphate and high in potassium, copper and selenium.[8]

MAY BE CONFUSED WITH A number of very closely related introduced plants grouped together under one name because it is so hard to distinguish between them. There are also many Australian native species *R. hillii*, *R. parvifolius* and *R. rosifolius*.

FURTHER READING Antioxidant, antimicrobial and neutrophil-modulating activities of herbal extracts.[10] *Rubus fruticosus* (blackberry) use as an herbal medicine.[10a] Antiviral effects of blackberry extract against herpes simplex virus type 1.[11]

BLACKBERRY NIGHTSHADE

Garden Nightshade, Nastergal (S. Africa)

Solanum nigrum

DISTRIBUTION Native to Europe, North Africa and Asia and now naturalized all over the world in temperate and tropical regions. Naturalized throughout Australia.

HABITAT A variable species having many varieties and forms. Common weed of gardens, wasteland and cultivation.

DESCRIPTION

Short-lived shrub up to 1 m (3 ft 3 in) high, erect, branched and mostly hairless.

LEAVES Oval, alternate with wavy margins.

FLOWERS In groups of six to eight hanging from a common stalk. White, five petals with yellow anthers.

FRUIT/SEED Green when immature to dull black or purple-black fleshy berry when ripe, containing many flattened yellow seeds. Fruits ripen in summer.

USES

EDIBLE/OTHER Blackberry nightshade berries taste like a cross between licorice and tomato although sometimes they taste unpleasant – avoid these berries. ONLY EAT RIPE BERRIES. Cases of toxicity have occurred when children have eaten green, unripe berries. This weed grows prolifically at my place and I regularly eat the berries and spend some time collecting the small but numerous berries to make jam. In South Africa in the Orange Free State 'Nastergal' jams are popular at farm stalls. Leaves are eaten like spinach.

MEDICINAL I make an ointment from the leaves and berries in the warmer months when the fruits are mature. Excellent for cold sores, shingles, sore lips, first stages of acne, ringworm, neuralgia, impetigo and dry scaly skin. In Ayurvedic medicine, this herb is used for skin diseases, scabies, eczema, psoriasis, as a laxative, aphrodisiac, for fluid

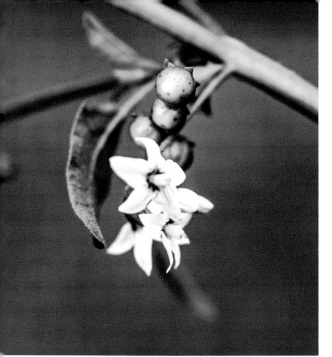 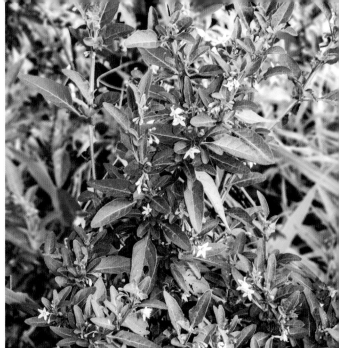

problems, jaundice, diarrhea and eye ailments. Other uses include for stomach ache, female ailments and liver disorders. In South Africa an infusion of the leaves is used for fevers, malaria, headaches, dysentery, diarrhea, as a sedative, wound wash, on ulcers, infected rashes and bites. Also useful to sooth hemorrhoids, varicosities and bruises. I've made a tasty gargle from berries with brandy and honey for a sore throat.

FARM/ENVIR. Worst weed in Australia for intensive agriculture. It grows with tomatoes, peas and numerous other crops and is a host for numerous nematodes, fungi, viruses and pests. Easy to eradicate in the early stages. Numerous plants grow on our property and are a host to pests that attack the potatoes. However, I grow this vegetable early in the season and when the pests have decimated my Blackberry nightshade plants my potatoes are finished. Keep livestock out of infested fields as green berries are toxic. In Ayurvedic medicine, the root is mixed with pepper and ginger then fed to cows to reduce gas formation in the stomach. Indicates soil is fertile if numerous healthy plants are growing together.

MAY BE CONFUSED WITH Deadly Nightshade (*Atropa belladonna*), rarely found in Australia and a different looking plant. Glossy Nightshade (*S. Americanum*) which has bigger, glossy black berries and similar medicinal uses.

FURTHER READING Antiproliferative effect of *Solanum nigrum* on human lukemic cell lines.[12] Studies on the molluscicidal and larvicidal properties of *Solanum nigrum* L. leaves in 70% ethanol extract.[13]

WARNING Green berries are toxic, contain alkaloid solanine.

BORAGE

Bee Bread, Starflower

Borago officinalis

DISTRIBUTION Native to Mediterranean region and now widespread throughout the world. Naturalized in southern Australia.

HABITAT Grown as a herb or as an ornament in gardens and readily seeds into wasteland, bushland, cultivation and pastures.

DESCRIPTION

Annual or biennial herb that branches out and grows leggy as it matures. Hairy, hollow stems up to 70 cm (2 ft 3 in) in height.

LEAVES Oval, alternate, rough leaves being hairy on both sides.

FLOWERS Numerous bright blue and occasionally pink, star-like flowers with black anthers in the center. Flowers grow on the end of stems and droop. Flowers spring/summer.

FRUIT/SEED Small green, hairy capsules containing black seeds. Readily self-sows.

USES

EDIBLE/OTHER Leaves have a salty cucumber flavor that I find, if well chopped and added to salads, give a pleasant flavor. Use fresh leaves and stems in cooked dishes. Add to Pimms and white wine based drinks. Flowers make a lovely garnish, freeze in ice blocks, add to vegetable and fruit salads or candy the flowers to decorate cakes. Refreshing tea made from leaves and flowers. Important source of nectar for bees. Dye from blue flowers used to color vinegars and white wines.

MEDICINAL Romans infused leaves in wine to relieve depression and improve mood. Used to relieve melancholy and an excellent herb as a tonic, helping restore adrenaline. Especially good after using cortisone and steroids. Take as tea, extract or use in your juice. Also good for fevers, as a diuretic, soothes sore throats, increases mother's milk supply,

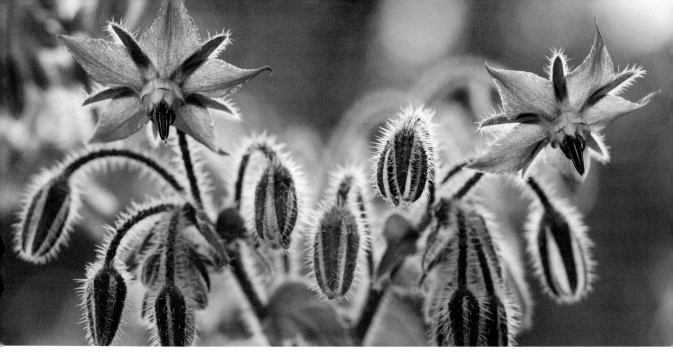

for inflammation, an antioxidant and good for memory. Externally soothes irritated skin, varicose veins and hemorrhoids. Seeds are crushed and an oil called 'Starflower' is commercially produced. High in GLA, which is good for balancing hormones, helping with PMT and blood pressure. Sadly, I can no longer sell this herb for internal use due to government legislation in Australia. Very controversial and banned as it contains the same alkaloid as Comfrey. There is no ban on usage at home and starflower oil is not affected.

FARM/ENVIR. I've grown a lot of Borage not just for the culinary and medicinal qualities but also for the bees. Great companion to strawberries and it's the best herb to break up clay. Stock will eat this plant and it's excellent for milk production. Excellent compost material. Popular in permaculture farming. Borage is an environmental weed in Victoria and a minor weed elsewhere.

MAY BE CONFUSED WITH Viper's Bugloss (*Echium vulgare* L.) which has narrow leaves and tubular flowers with four protruding stamens and one smaller. Paterson's Curse (*Echium plantagineum* L.), which has large purplish-blue flowers with two protruding stamens and three smaller.

FURTHER READING Protective effects of *Borago officinalis* extract on Amyloid Ð-Peptide (25–35) – induced memory impairment in male rats: a behavioral study.[15] Extraction of antioxidants from borage (*Borago officinalis* L.) leaves – optimization by response surface method and application in oil-in-water emulsions.[16]

WARNING Government legislation in Australia prohibits the sale of this plant for internal use. Hairs on the plant may cause skin irritation.

BOXTHORN

African Boxthorn

Lycium ferocissimum

DISTRIBUTION Native of South Africa and now naturalized in America and scattered in Europe and Asia. Naturalized throughout Australia.

HABITAT Found in pastures, roadsides, wastelands, forest edges and neglected farming land.

DESCRIPTION

Intricately branched shrub up to 5 m (16 ft) high with long, rigid branches, lateral branches ending in a stout spine.

LEAVES Fleshy, bright green, clustered, mostly oval.

FLOWERS White with purplish throat, five petals and fragrant. Flowers mainly in summer.

FRUIT/SEED Dull orange-red, egg-shaped berry. Contains about 70 dull yellow seeds. Fruit eaten by birds and foxes.

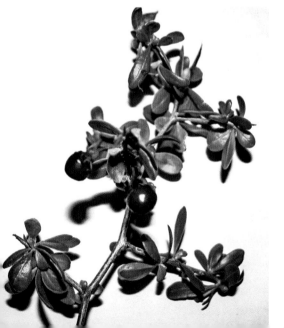
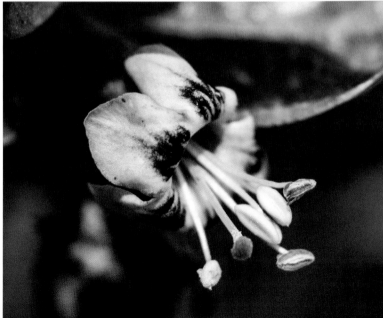

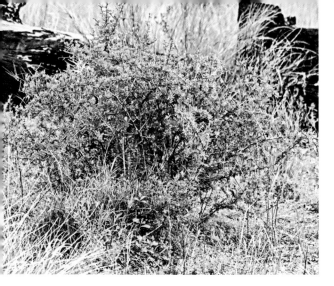
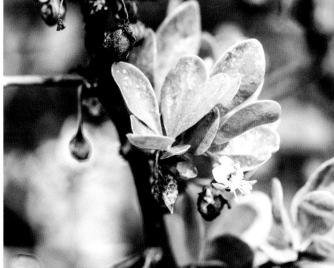

USES

EDIBLE/OTHER Boxthorn is in the Solanaceae family, which is renowned for having both edible and toxic species. I have collected these berries (beware of spines) and made a very tasty jam. Sometimes when eaten fresh they have a sweet tomato flavor, other times they are not palatable. When berries dry on the bush, they taste like sultanas. Ensure you eat only ripe berries. In health food stores, Wolfberry and Boxthorn berries are often mixed with Goji – hard to tell the difference as closely related. Good honey plant. In arid Australia Aborigines ate fruit of *Lycium austral* (a close relative).

MEDICINAL Related to other *Lycium* species such as Goji berries (*L. barbarum*) and Wolfberry (*L. sinensis*), which have medicinal usage. Claimed to prolong life, tonic against cancer, aphrodisiac, relieve aches and pains and improves immune system. Tests have shown it is a good antioxidant and may lower blood pressure, cholesterol and blood sugar levels.

FARM/ENVIR. Brought to Australia in 1800s as a hedge. A noxious weed which forms dense thickets that impede stock from reaching water. Also harbors foxes and rabbits. Difficult to eradicate. On the positive side, if kept in check it makes an excellent windbreak and hedgerow even for poultry, birds and wildlife, all of whom are safe in its thorny enclosure. Not normally grazed by animals due to its thorns. Goats will graze on this plant although potentially toxic.

MAY BE CONFUSED WITH Chinese Boxthorn or Goji berries (*Lycium barbarum*) which have thin, ovate leaves and shorter leafless branches reduced to a spine or no spine. Naturalized in Eastern Australia.

FURTHER READING Extraction of carotenoids from *Lycium ferocissimum* fruits for cotton dyeing.[17]

WARNING Contains the toxic alkaloid solanine.

BRACKEN

Australian Bracken, Western Bracken

Pleridium esculentum, Pleridium aquilinum (and subspecies)

DISTRIBUTION Australian Bracken grows throughout Australia, New Zealand and Pacific Islands. Western Bracken is naturalized throughout the world. Naturalized in southern and eastern Australia. Some authors believe that there is one world species (*P. aquilinum*) with many subspecies and varieties. Controversial.

HABITAT Serious weed of pastures, roadsides, disturbed areas, watercourses and recreational areas.

DESCRIPTION

Perennial fern 150 cm (5 ft) high with a complex underground stem system (rhizomes) which can become a vast network which gives rise to new shoots.

LEAVES Fiddleheads start bright green and coiled expanding to emerald green, deeply-divided leathery fronds (leaves) on robust brown stalks. Brown as it matures and dies off.

FRUIT/SEED Spores in late summer/autumn.

USES

EDIBLE/OTHER Fiddleheads eaten throughout the world especially in Japan where it is a delicacy. Picked in spring, eaten fresh or preserved by salting, pickling and drying. Fronds and rhizomes used to brew beer and rhizomes ground as a substitute for arrowroot. In addition, American Indians and Australian Aborigines used the ground and roasted rhizomes as a flour. As it has carcinogenic and mutagenic properties, it is best to eat minimally. Contains a toxic substance called ptaquiloside, which is water soluble and partially destroyed by boiling. Therefore, always soak in salty water and cook well before eating. In the Middle Ages, bracken was so valuable it was used to pay rents. Used for thatch, bedding, soap and as fuel for quick fire. Used in the glass industry. Rhizomes tan leather and dye wool yellow.

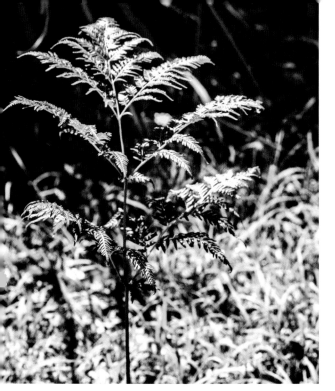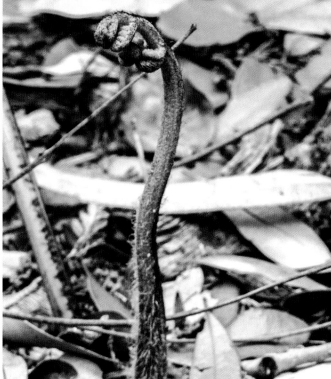

MEDICINAL Powdered rhizomes effective against parasitic worms. American Indians used rhizomes as a remedy for bronchitis and South African tribes used the ground and roasted meal to treat diarrhea and stomach ache. Tincture of the root is used in wine for rheumatism, boil the whole plant for TB. Young shoots are diuretic and cooling. Potential source of insecticides.[18] Rub young stems on insect bites. I find they work great on nettle stings.

FARM/ENVIR. Competes with other crops and pastures, extracts from dry fronds have shown that they inhibit other plants. Toxic to sheep, pigs, horses and cattle if eaten in large quantities (although they usually avoid grazing the stiff fronds). Eaten mainly by goats. Green fronds and rhizomes very toxic. If pigs are used to dig up bracken to eradicate it, give them Vitamin B1 injection. Burning, plowing and replacing with pasture or slashing in winter helps to control growth.[19] However, it makes excellent potash (burn bracken), which is high in potassium to fertilize your garden; good green crop; compost material to improve soil fertility. Potential as biofuel. Use rhizomes to worm livestock. Indicates soil very low in calcium, high in potassium and zinc with low humus and moisture, good drainage, sandy and presence of aluminum.[8]

FURTHER READING Unites States Forest Service plants database.[18] Immunosuppressive effects of *Pteridium aquilinum* enhance susceptibility to urethane-induced lung carcinogenesis.[20]

WARNING Research reveals the link with various cancers in humans and animals. Potentially toxic.

BRASSICA

Indian Mustard (*B. juncea*), **Wild Turnip** (*B. rapa*), **Twiggy Turnip** (*B. fruticulosa*), **Mediterranean Turnip** (*B. tournefortii*)

DISTRIBUTION Indian Mustard native to Asia and naturalized in southern and eastern Australia; Wild Turnip native to Europe and naturalized in southern and eastern Australia; Twiggy Turnip native to southern Europe and North Africa and naturalized mainly in Victoria and eastern New South Wales; Mediterranean Turnip native to the Mediterranean region and naturalized throughout Australia. All four now widespread in temperate regions throughout the world.

HABITAT Found in cultivation, disturbed areas, roadsides, pastures, wastelands and neglected farmland.

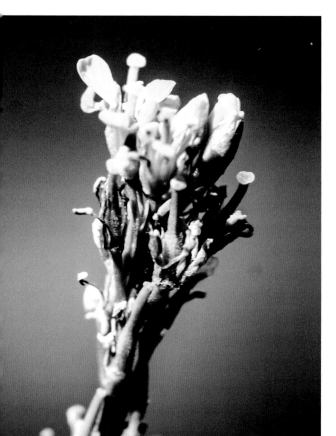

DESCRIPTION

Annual or biennial herb in the cabbage family.

LEAVES Brassica species produce a basal rosette of leaves before their stems elongate and produce flowers.

FLOWERS Yellow with four sepals and four petals diagonally disposed looking like a cross.

FRUIT/SEED Distinctive fruiting pod characterizes the family. Pods may end in a pointed beak. Fruits of this genus have divided walls, which break into separate pieces (valves) to release seeds.

DIFFERENCES BETWEEN SPECIES Indian Mustard has stalked hairless leaves along upper stems and pods 2.5–6 cm (1–2.4 in) long with seedless beaks. Wild Turnip is the wild form of the cultivated turnip but its root is less swollen. Distinguished by its stem clasping upper leaves and pods 4–6.5 cm (1.6–2.6 in) long with seedless beaks. Twiggy Turnip is similar to Indian Mustard except the beak is short and blunt with one or two seeds. Mediterranean Turnip with its long taproot has bristly pinnate leaves that lie flat on the ground and is the most aggressive and vigorous of the brassicas.

USES

EDIBLE/OTHER Brassica family are an edible species. I tasted my first mustard leaf in the middle of summer when the plant was mature and it was extremely pungent – brought tears to my eyes. Pick leaves, shoots and flower buds when young and add them to salads or your cooking. If eating older leaves you may need to chop and cook them well to reduce the pungency. You can use the dried seeds just like mustard seeds. A good quality oil obtained from the seeds of Black, White and Indian Mustard has been used for cooking for thousands of years. Canola oil or rapeseed oil (mustard family) is a highly refined mustard oil in commercial production.

MEDICINAL Mustard essential oil used in India, Bangladesh and other countries for cleansing, stimulating and revitalizing of the body. The oil you buy for cooking has many health benefits. Mustard seed plasters are an old remedy to relieve backache, sciatica pain and to relieve congestion of a cold. Do not overuse these plasters, as they will cause blisters and severe pain. I tried using a mustard poultice on my chest before I understood about this herb and received severe burns. At the time, I was unaware of the correct procedure in using this strong poultice. Ayurvedic, Unani and Sidha medicine use Indian and Wild Turnip leaves in soups to treat bladder, inflammation and hemorrhage. Seeds are used to treat abscesses, headaches, colds, fever, flu, arthritis, tumor, foot ache, sores, lumbago, rheumatism and stomach disorders. The oil is used on skin eruptions and ulcers.

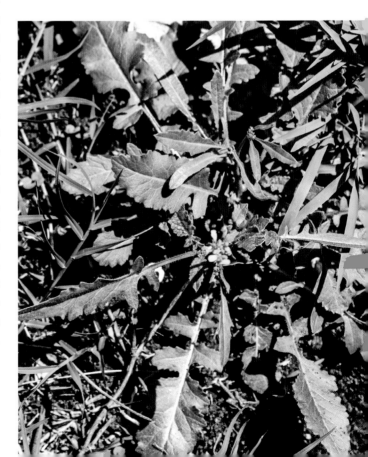

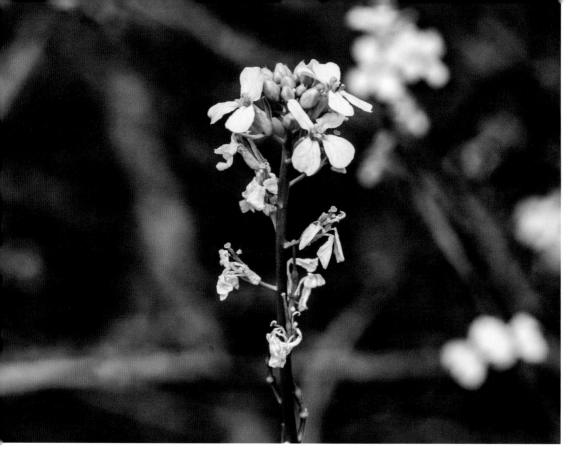

FARM/ENVIR. Some of the wild Brassicas such as the Indian Mustard and Wild Turnip are used as fodder crops. Especially when eaten young these plants are very nutritious. Mustards are good pest control agents and also deters nematodes. Use as a green crop and plough in for better growth of Solanaceae plants such as potatoes, tomatoes and other crops. These plants grow prolifically when earth is compacted and produce alkaline secretions on the roots that sweeten acid soil. They can absorb excessive salts and return them in organic form. In fact, mustards collect salt in larger quantities than other plants. In Ayurvedic, Unani and Sidha medicine roots of the Indian mustard are given to cows to promote milk, and crushed seeds promote reproduction. Wild Turnip is given to cows after delivery for removal of placenta. Leaf juice also used for wounds. Indian Brassica indicates in the soil is very low calcium and manganese, very high in potassium, magnesium and chloride. Low humus, bacteria, moisture, high in salt with good drainage and hard crust.[8]

FURTHER READING Rai (*B. Juncea*) significantly prevented the development of insulin resistance in rats fed fructose-enriched diet.[21]

WARNING Eaten in large quantities, the seeds in particular have sulfurous compounds that can be toxic to stock.

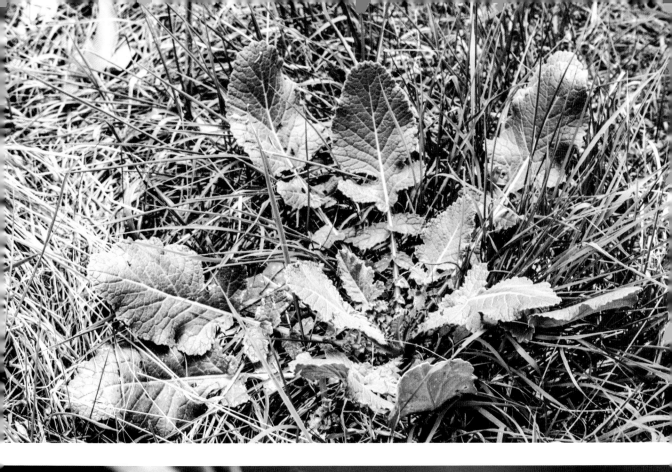

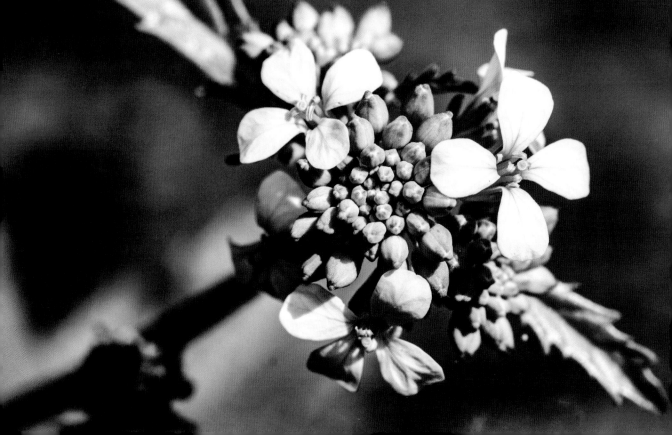

BUGLE

Ajuga, Common or Creeping Bugle, Carpenter's Herb

Ajuga reptans

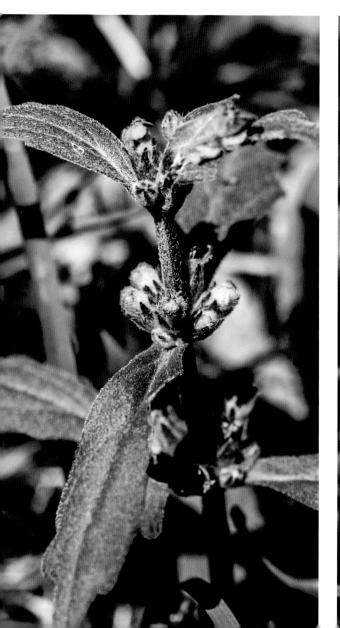
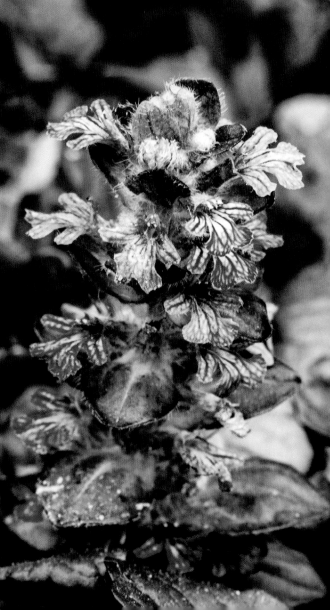

DISTRIBUTION Native to Europe now widespread. Grows in south-east Australia.

HABITAT Cultivated as an ornamental ground cover and has escaped onto roadsides, along creeks and other damp sites.

DESCRIPTION

Perennial low growing herb with stems that spread across the surface of the ground. It has erect flowering stems 10–35 cm (4–14 in) tall.

LEAF Oval, purple-green leaves with wavy margins. Start as a rosette then flowering stem appears.

FLOWERS On the end of the square, hairy stem, six to twelve whorls of blue flowers appear in early-to-late summer.

FRUIT/SEED Mature fruit splits into four chambers full of seeds.

USES

EDIBLE/OTHER Leaves and young shoots are edible. It makes a healthy, bitter tea, just add other herbs such as peppermint and lemon to improve the flavor.

MEDICINAL Formerly used to stop hemorrhages (Carpenter's Herb) as it is a good astringent. Also useful for coughs and ulcers. Externally used as an ointment or infused oil for wounds, bruises and tumors. Seventeenth century herbalist Nicholas Culpeper suggested that it is a cure for hangovers. I've drunk the bitter tea for a cough; it was helpful.

FARM/ENVIR. Naturalized in Tasmania where it is now an environmental weed. Introduced in 1978 and spread quickly. Forms thick mats which threaten native ground cover. A minor weed growing in dark, shady spots where pasture does not grow. Not poisonous to stock. Easy and hardy to grow and its foliage is always ornamental. Much loved by a variety of butterflies.

MAY BE CONFUSED WITH New horticultural varieties such as *A. purpurea* and *A. variegate* grown as ornamentals. No medicinal qualities.

FURTHER READING Ethnopharmacology of the plants of genus *Ajuga* [22]

BULRUSH

Broadleaf Cumbungi, Southern Cattail and Broadleaf Cattail

Typha orientalis, *Typha domingensis* and *Typha latifolia*

DISTRIBUTION Broadleaf Cumbungi is native to Australia, New Zealand, Eastern and South-East Asia. Naturalized in southern, eastern and coastal areas of Australia; Southern Cattail often confused with *T. angustifolia* is worldwide and naturalized throughout Australia; Broadleaf Cattail is native to Europe and North America and now widespread, naturalized in south-eastern Australia.

HABITAT Invasive plant growing in marshy wet areas, beside dams, rivers and streams. It is a major weed of irrigation systems and rice.

DESCRIPTION

Erect, reed-like perennials 1.5–4 m (4 ft 9 in–13 ft) high with rhizomes and cylindrical stems.

LEAVES Pithy leaf blades linear up to 1 m (3 ft 3 in) long.

FLOWERS Spring/summer erect spike forms of tightly packed clusters of single-sex flowers (male above).

FRUIT/SEED When pollen released, male flower withers and female gives rise to tiny fruits with numerous silky hairs (down) around each seed to produce familiar furry, brown, cylindrical seed heads.

DIFFERENCES BETWEEN SPECIES Broadleaf Cumbungi has a female spike 1–4 cm (0.4–1.6 in) in diameter and may or may not be separate from the male spike. Southern Cattail female spike is narrower, less than 2 cm (0.8 in) in diameter, longer and separate from male spike. Broadleaf Cattail female spike is darker in color with no bracts and not separate from male spike.

USES

EDIBLE/USES Survivalist plant — no other plant is so widespread with so many edible and practical uses. Nutty tasting pollen makes a nutritious protein rich bread; small white shoots cooked like asparagus and rhizomes are full of starch so make good flat cakes. Young female flower spikes when boiled while green, and tiny seeds, are both edible. Leaves can be used for weaving, roof thatching and making baskets. Aborigines made string from the rhizomes after extracting the starch. The down is used as tinder to start fires; packed around wounds to staunch bleeding and can be packed into rags as absorbent pad during menstruation. My class took hours to extract the edible starch to make a small edible hot cake, which we cut into 12 tiny pieces and savored! We then tried to make a respectable piece of string with not much luck.

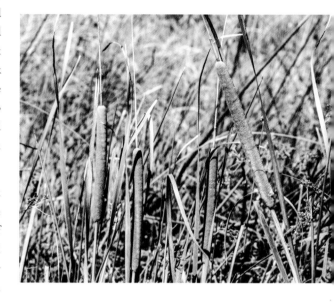

MEDICINAL All over the world, different cultures used bulrushes as medicine. The traditional uses are varied. Broadleaf Cumbungi root used as an astringent and diuretic; Southern Cattail pollen used for period problems, stomach problems and strains, externally for skin inflammation and wounds; Broadleaf cattail poultice made from roots applied to wounds, boils, sores and infections. In Africa tea made from the roots is used for dysentery and diarrhea.

FARM/ENVIR. Bulrushes protect wildlife and help with erosion, good for wastewater treatment and when burnt make a good fertilizer. However, its best use is for industrial site remediation as it tolerates heavy metals and has the ability to reduce sulfates and heavy metals from mine tailings. Good fodder and forage for stock. Bulrushes will choke streams, stop cattle getting to water and interfere with fishing and water transport. Difficult to eradicate, however, short-term control best by cutting, burning and grazing.[23] Indicates soil high in magnesium, low in humus, bacteria and moisture with hardpan and poor drainage.[8]

FURTHER READING Effects of EDTA on lead uptake by *Typha orientalis* Presl.: a new lead-accumulating species in southern China.[24] (*T. orientalis*) The ability of *Typha domingensis* to accumulate and tolerate high concentrations of Cr, Ni, and Zn.[25] (*T. domingensis*)

WARNING Some authors warn of toxins in Bulrushes for stock that eat large quantities.

BURDOCK

Cocklebur, Thorny Burr, Greater Burdock

Arctium lappa

DISTRIBUTION Native to Eurasia and now widespread in the cooler parts of the world. In Australia naturalized in New South Wales and Victoria and a noxious weed in Tasmania.

HABITAT Moist, fertile soil of roadways, waste places and pastures.

DESCRIPTION

Stout handsome biennial or perennial herb up to 2 m (6 ft 6 in) tall with fine hairy stems when in flower.

LEAVES Large heart-shaped to oval with fine down on under side. Leaves on flowering stalks smaller.

FLOWERS Like thistle flowers with purple petals sitting softly atop stiff, globular bracts covered with spiny hooks.

FRUIT/SEED Flowers turn into a burr with brownish-grey wrinkled seeds.

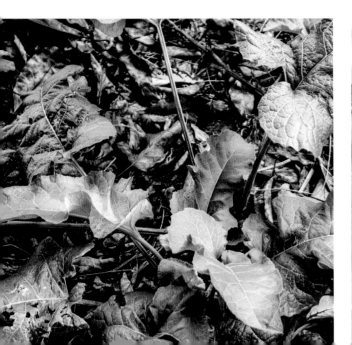
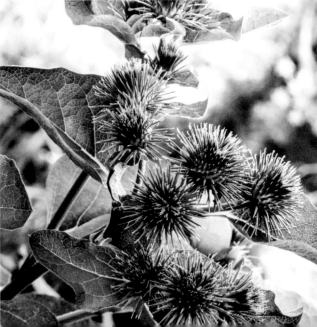

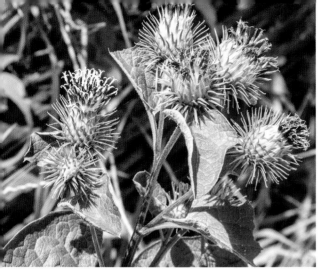
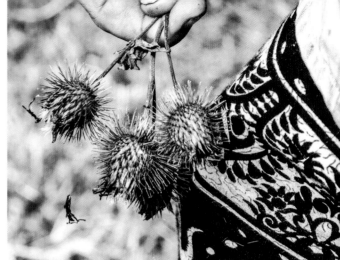

USES

EDIBLE/OTHER Leaves eaten only when very young (bitter and tough when older). Young stalks peeled, eaten in salads or cooked like asparagus. Use only first year roots (older roots tough and stringy); contains inulin, a dietary fiber; popular in Japan (called 'gobo').

MEDICINAL A renowned alterative herb that cleanses and purifies the system acting via the liver. Especially good for dry skin conditions such as psoriasis and acne and eczema. Leaves, seeds and roots are used. Western herbal medicine extracts are made from the roots and I use this preparation to help many of my clients with dry skin problems. Other uses are respiratory problems, boils, gout, rheumatism, cancer, diabetes and externally for ulcers, tumors and inflammation.

FARM/ENVIR. This plant is becoming a more serious weed in agriculture due to non-till farming. It is easily controlled by cultivation. The burrs attach themselves to any animal that passes, spreading them over a wider area. It affects the quality of sheep's wool and goat hair. I remember my dog getting them attached to its tail and legs, sticking these parts together – very distressing. Burdock grown commercially for roots is dug up in the first year, before flowering. Indicates soil low in calcium, very high in potassium, high in magnesium, manganese, boron and selenium. Low humus, bacteria and hardpan.[8]

MAY BE CONFUSED WITH Common or Lesser Burdock (*A. minus*) has similar habitat and properties to Greater Burdock. Difference is that Lesser Burdock has clusters of smaller flowers and basal leaves with hollow stems.

FURTHER READING Anti-inflammatory and radical scavenge effects of *Arctium lappa*.[26] Hepatoprotective effects of *Arctium lappa* Linne on liver injuries induced by chronic ethanol consumption and potentiated by carbon tetrachloride.[27]

WARNING Contact dermatitis with sensitive individuals and avoid if allergic to the daisy family.

BUSY LIZZIE

Impatiens, Garden Balsam

Impatiens walleriana

DISTRIBUTION Native to tropical Africa now established worldwide. Naturalized on the eastern coast of Australia.

HABITAT Grown in gardens for its color and once established hard to eradicate. Seeds have germinated in bushland, along watercourses and around habitation.

DESCRIPTION

In frost-free areas, this colorful plant is perennial but often grown as an annual in gardens. Plants grow up to 1 m (3 ft 3 in) high with succulent translucent stems.

LEAVES Mid-green, fleshy, oval leaves spirally arranged.

FLOWERS Appear in pairs or threes at leaf stem junction on top part of plant. Five petals 3 cm (1.2 in) in diameter in shades of pink, rose, red and occasionally white.

FRUIT/SEED Smooth greenish capsule. Ripe fruits explode ejecting small brownish seeds.

USES

EDIBLE/OTHER Sweet flowers are edible, add to salads and fancy drinks; I love freezing them in ice blocks then dropping them in a drink.

MEDICINAL Ayurvedic, Unani and Sidha medicine. Used internally for circulation, as a tonic, for pain, respiratory and fluid problems. Externally used on clean wounds, burns and skin problems.

FARM/ENVIR. Grows in remnant bush and shady, wetland margins. Found in National Parks displacing natural vegetation especially along watercourses. Brittle stems easily broken and carried downstream by floodwaters. Colonies on forest margins displacing native ferns especially around waterfalls. I find colonies of these bright flowering plants in Queensland on the forest margins. Attracts butterflies and fodder for goats.

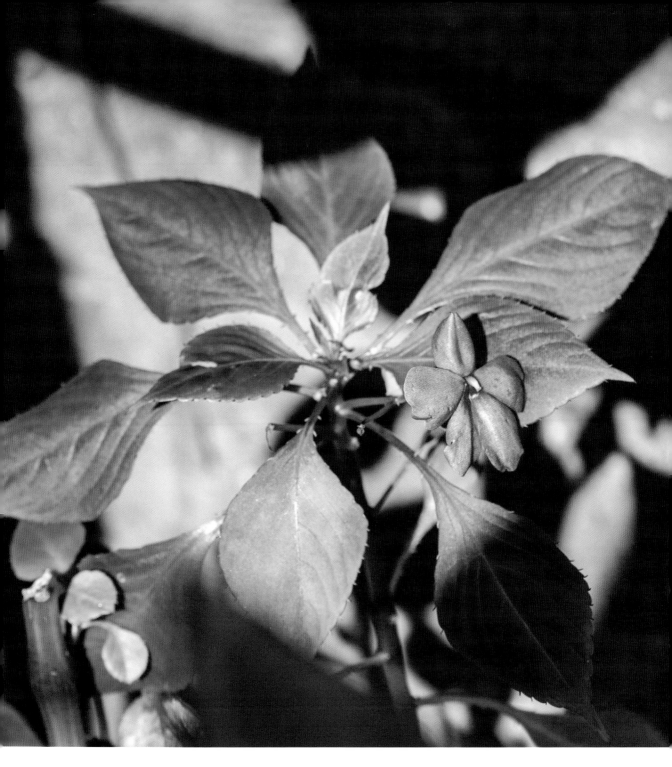

FURTHER READING Edible flowers – a new promising source of mineral elements in human nutrition.[28] Chelator effects on bioconcentration and translocation of cadmium by hyperaccumulators.[29]

CALIFORNIAN POPPY

Golden Poppy

Eschscholzia californica

DISTRIBUTION Native to USA and Mexico (State flower of California), now a widespread garden escapee in Mediterranean climates. Naturalized to south-eastern and south-western Australia.

HABITAT A pretty weed of riverbanks and roadsides often on the fringe of country towns.

DESCRIPTION

Annual or perennial 13–152 cm (5 in–4 ft 10 in) tall easily recognized with its bright flowers.

LEAVES Bluish-green in color and deeply dissected.

FLOWERS Solitary on long stems, silky textured with four petals, yellow-orange in color. Flowers in warmer months, closing at night.

FRUIT/SEEDS Cylindrical ribbed capsule when split releases numerous small dark seeds.

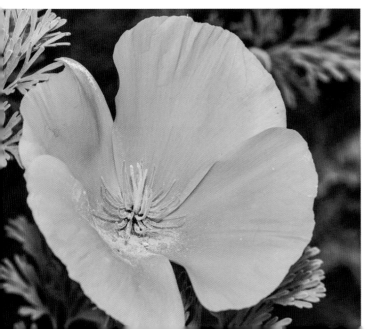

USES

EDIBLE/OTHER Leaves boiled and roasted before being eaten by the North American Indians despite the bitter flavor.

MEDICINAL Closely related to true poppies, which have sedative properties. Western herbalists use this plant for its painkilling and sedentary effects, helps with sleeplessness, anxiety and nerve

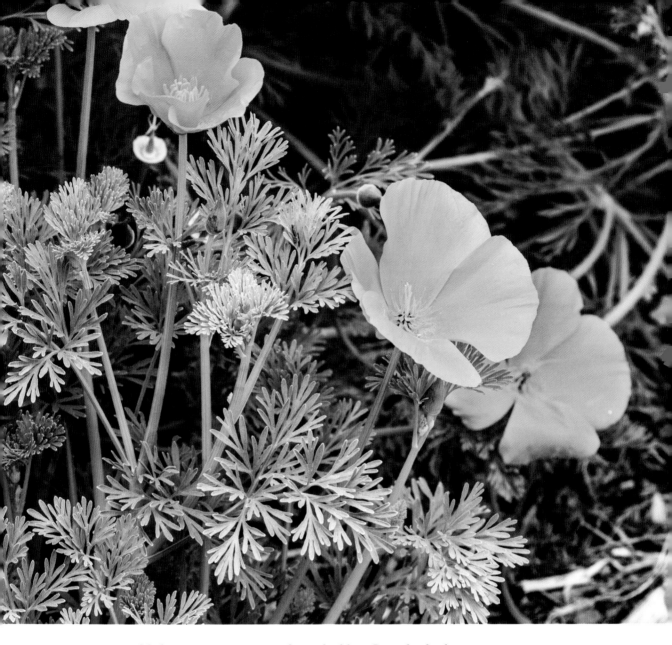

pain. Made into tinctures, capsules and tablets. I use this herb as an extract in my practice and find it very useful if people cannot sleep due to pain. Latex used for toothache and whole plant used to stun fish.

FARM/ENVIR. Important plant to have in your garden or paddock as it attracts a wide range of useful insects who love the vibrant and pollen-rich flowers. I love seeing them growing wild in my sister's place in Tasmania.

FURTHER READING Sedative and anxiolytic properties.[30] Another experiment with mice induced peripheral analgesic effects.[31]

CALTROP

Cathead, Puncture Vine, Bindii, Goathead

Tribulus terrestris

DISTRIBUTION Native to the Mediterranean region and now naturalized in tropical and subtropical regions. Grows throughout Australia.

HABITAT Gardens, recreational areas, crops, vineyards, pastoral land and wasteland. Will grow even in desert climates and poor soil.

DESCRIPTION

Branching, prostate annual or perennial with stems up to 2 m (6 ft 6 in) long and a woody taproot. Can cover large areas.

LEAVES Four to eight pairs of unequal, oblong-to-oval leaflets. Upper surface dark green and paler underneath.

FLOWERS Five bright yellow petals, borne singly. Flowers in the warmer months.

FRUIT/SEED Star-shaped burr comprising a cluster of five segments each covered with short, hard points. Each segment has one to five seeds.

USES

EDIBLE/OTHER Used for medicinal purposes only.

MEDICINAL This plant is used in folk medicine in China, Bulgaria and South Africa for a variety of reproductive conditions such as infertility and sexual impotence, decreased libido as well as for muscle strength, cystitis, kidney stones, edemas, cardiovascular diseases and general health. Also for gout and cough. The leaf and stem from Eastern Europe is used in Bulgaria where it is standardized and many authors and companies now sell only this extract. However, there is a great deal of research on *Tribulus* fruit from India also showing good results. Research is ongoing.

FARM/ENVIR. This plant will grow over large areas and the sharp spines on the dry fruit

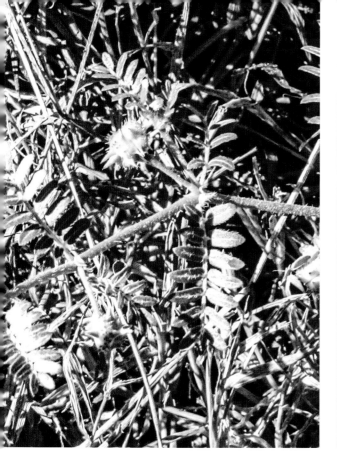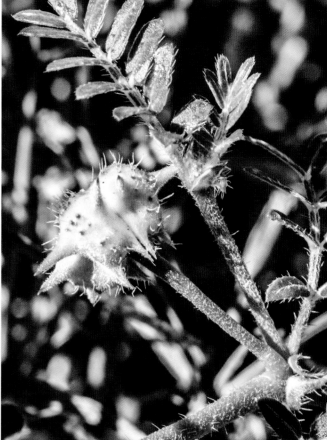

hamper stock handling and are a nuisance in recreation areas. Avoid grazing on infested paddocks. Young sheep are especially sensitive. It may injure stock's feet and contaminates wool. There is a native insect and mite used overseas for biological control of this plant. It was growing all over one of our flats where people camp, so I cleared this area by daily hoeing, and removing before it flowered. Took me weeks but it has not returned. Very unpleasant on the feet and will puncture bicycle and lawn mower tyres. Indicates soils low in calcium, very low in phosphate and very high in potassium, high in magnesium and other minerals. Low moisture, good drainage and sandy soil.[8]

MAY BE CONFUSED WITH Yellow vine (*T. micrococcus*) which is spineless and occurs in New South Wales and Queensland.

FURTHER READING Evaluation of the aphrodisiac activity of *Tribulus terrestris* L. In sexually sluggish male albino rats.[32] The hormonal effects of *Tribulus terrestris* and its role in the management of male erectile dysfunction—an evaluation using primates, rabbit and rat.[33] Chronic Administration of *Tribulus terrestris* L. extract improves cardiac function and attenuates myocardial infarction in rats.[35]

WARNING Toxic to stock when eaten in large amounts. May cause photosensitization, staggers and nitrate poisoning.

CENTAURY

Common or European Centaury and Centaury Spike

Centaurium erythraea and *Centaurium spicatum*

DISTRIBUTION *C. erythraea* is native to Europe and now widespread in wetter areas of Australia. *C. spicatum* is native to Australia and widespread.

HABITAT *C. erythraea* likes damper habitats in pastures, cultivation and woodland areas where it competes with native ground species. *C spicatum* is found in pastures, grasslands and wasteland.

DESCRIPTION

These annual/biennial plants are up to 50 cm (1 ft 6 in) tall. Both species are very similar except that *C. spicatum* has less numerous flower heads, which are loose, leafy and can occur on the lower part of the plant.

LEAVES Opposite leaves are stalkless, oblon,g tapering at both ends.

FLOWERS Five petals, mainly pink in color. Flowers spring/summer and dies down after seeding.

FRUIT/SEEDS Minute seeds in cylindrical capsules.

USES

EDIBLE/OTHER These flowers have a bitter taste and bitters are very good for the digestive system so make them part of your diet. When flowering I eat a few flower heads as I collect them to dry or juice for tincture.

MEDICINAL The bitter principle of these plants makes them good for digestive problems as well as a tonic. The more researched *C. erythraea* is used to stimulate appetite (drink a cup of the infusion half an hour before meals), helps digestion, heartburn, good for worming and externally the fresh herb is used as a poultice for wounds and sores. Culpeper says 'Tis very wholesome but not very toothsome'.

FARM/ENVIR. Avoided by animals due to its bitterness. A pretty little plant, which I enjoy seeing in the warmer months with its distinctive pink flowers, usually a weed of minor significance.

FURTHER READING Experimental diuretic effects of *Rosmarinus officinalis* and *Centaurium erythraea*.[35] Hepatoprotective activity of *Centaurium erythraea* on acetaminophen-induced hepatotoxicity in rats (protects liver).[36] Antioxidant activity of *Centaurium erythraea* infusion.[37]

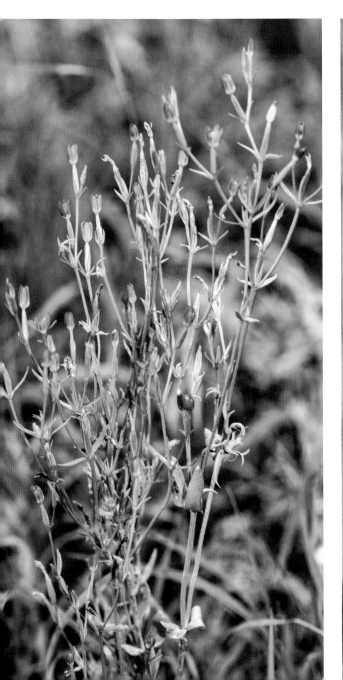
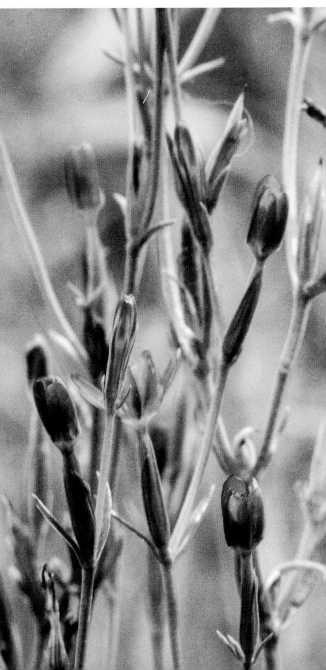

CHICKWEED

Starweed

Stellaria media

DISTRIBUTION Native to Europe now worldwide. Naturalized in south-eastern Australia.

HABITAT Common weed of shaded gardens, liking moist, rich soils. Found in orchards, pastures and in crops.

DESCRIPTION

Delicate low growing annual distinguished by a line of small white hairs, which run up on one side of the stem, and changes sides between each pair of leaves. Stems have many branches that trail along the ground for some distance. Will grow all year round in cold climates but only in the cooler months in hot climates.

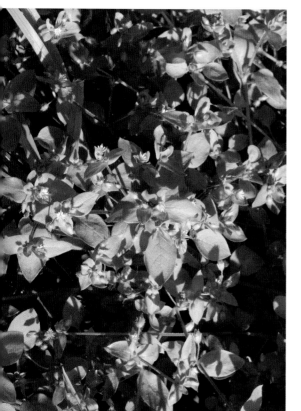

LEAVES Are green and luscious with an oval shape.

FLOWERS Tiny, star-like, single near upper leaves.

FRUIT/SEED Tiny seeds are contained in small capsules fitted with teeth and are dispersed in the wind.

USES

EDIBLE/OTHER Praise the day when you find this straggler in your garden as this is a neglected nutritious herb containing valuable potash salts, iron, antioxidants and other minerals. Seeds found in the ancient Tollund and Grauballe men show this herb has been eaten for thousands of years. Cut off young tops

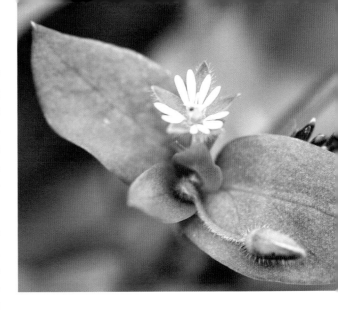

and eat them like sprouts in salads, put them in soups, stews, in your morning smoothie or juice, on your sandwich like lettuce, you can even make a whole salad based on this herb. I eat the young tops regularly in winter when I have only a few greens in the garden; it tastes rather similar to alfalfa sprouts.

MEDICINAL Held in great esteem by herbalists for all irritations of the skin. Think of this herb if skin is hot and itchy such as eczema, psoriasis, bites, nappy rash and other irritations. Has antiviral and antifungal properties. Also useful for cuts and wounds. I make an ointment for dry skin conditions and a cream for wet skin conditions, using only the fresh plant, with good results, especially in children with eczema. Also used as a poultice. Use the fresh herb internally for rheumatism, piles, catarrhal conditions of the lungs, kidneys and bladder. It is a soothing eye lotion. Poultices used for carbuncle, boils, abscesses and painful rheumatic joints. Popular for losing weight.[38] Indicates soil very low in magnesium and phosphate, very high in potassium, high in magnesium, iron and other minerals. Low humus, hard crust and presence of aluminum.[8]

FARM/ENVIR. This plant is an indicator that the land is fertile. Enjoyed by chickens, birds, pigs, rabbits, cows and horses. Sheep are indifferent and goats ignore it. Make an infused oil, ointment or poultice for irritations of the skin on all animals especially the 'summer itch'. Overseas the plant was encouraged to grow to increase fruit yield.

MAY BE CONFUSED WITH Petty Spurge (*Euphorbia peplus*) which is similar when younger but is distinguished by its white sap; Mouse Ear Chickweed (*Cerastium glomeratum*) which has sticky, hairy leaves; Scarlet Pimpernel (*Anagallis arvensis*) which has stalkless leaves and red or blue flowers.

FURTHER READING Quality assessment and antiobesity activity of *Stellaria media* (L.) Vill.[38] There are several articles on trialing Chickweed for its antiobesity activity and have favorable results using lyophilized juice or methanolic extract (tincture had poorer results). Anti-hepatitis B virus activity of Chickweed [*Stellaria media* (L.) Vill.] extracts in HepG2.2.15 cells.[39] A novel antifungal peptide from leaves of the weed *Stellaria media* L.[40]

WARNING Many authors state that Chickweed contains saponins so beware of consuming large amounts of this plant. However, Gibbs (1974) reported negative results in saponin tests on leaf material.[41]

CHICORY

Succory

Cichorium intybus

DISTRIBUTION Native to Europe and temperate Asia now established in temperate climates throughout the world. Naturalized in southern and eastern Australia.

HABITAT Common weed of roadsides and wasteland. Purposely introduced but like many wayside weeds escaped into the wild.

DESCRIPTION

Erect perennial 120 cm (3 ft 9 in) tall recognized by its tall, rigid, almost leafless stems covered in flowers. Has a long, stout taproot.

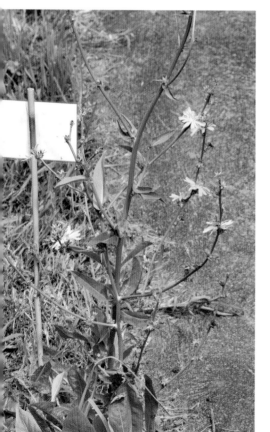

LEAVES Starts as a rosette of large leaves similar to Dandelion but slightly rougher with smaller stem leaves.

FLOWERS Distinct blue flowers in clusters of two or three borne on upper part of the stalk. Flowers open around midday and flower over the warmer months.

USES

EDIBLE/OTHER Chicory is renowned as a coffee substitute: dig up the root before flowering (otherwise it will be tough and stringy) and cut into large pieces; roast in the oven on a low heat until light brown inside, cool and grind and you will have a superior beverage to the commercial charred variety. Root also used as a substitute for parsnip. Young Chicory leaves have a bitter flavor similar

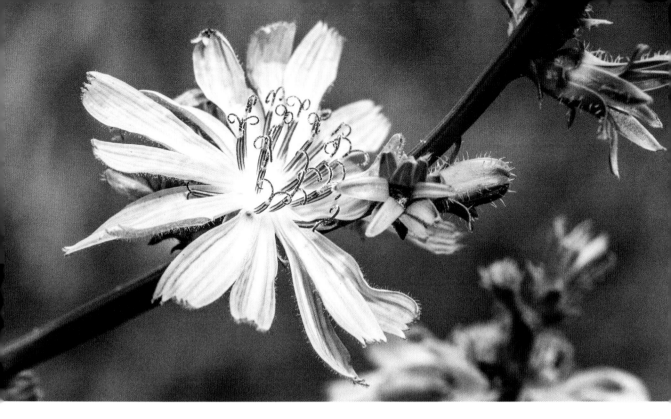

to the Witlof and Endive varieties and can be eaten raw in salads or cooked. A popular vegetable in some cultures. Flowers edible and used as garnish.

MEDICINAL Medicinally important plant of Eurasia and parts of Africa for centuries. Modern research has confirmed many of the folk remedies. Used for cancer of the uterus, tumors, antimicrobial, antimalarial, antidiabetic (containing 40% inulin, a dietary fiber), anti-inflammatory and antioxidant. Other uses are for pain, gallstones and liver, digestive problems and worming. Externally make an ointment for wound healing and bruises. A syrup is made from the bitter root as a tonic for infants.

FARM/ENVIR. Not an agricultural problem as animals will always graze on chicory. In Europe grown as a fodder crop: cow's milk may taste bitter but horses, sheep, rabbits and poultry thrive on this herb. Bees love the blue flowers. If you see a colony of healthy plants it is an indicator of good soil. Deep roots bring up nutrients and aerate the soil. There are colonies of Chicory plants beside the road that I enjoy as I drive to work and I grow many plants myself. I enjoy the flowers and use the leaves regularly. Indicates soil low in calcium and high in potassium, magnesium, zinc, boron and other minerals. Low humus and bacteria and a hard crust.[8]

FURTHER READING *Cichorium intybus:* traditional uses, phytochemistry, pharmacology, and toxicology.[42]

WARNING Member of the daisy family so avoid if sensitive.

CLIVERS

Cleavers, Goosegrass, Sticky Willie

Galium aparine

DISTRIBUTION Native of Europe and now spread to all temperate climates of the world. Naturalized in southern and eastern Australia.

HABITAT Creek banks, fields, roadsides, gardens, orchards, crops and forests. Prefers a moist site.

DESCRIPTION

Annual, sprawling, distinctive weed. Has a weakly climbing habit. Square stems are bristly and sticky having Velcro-like hooks on the angles of the stems, that attach to clothes, fur etc.

LEAVES Bristly, sprouting from stems in clusters of six to eight.

FLOWERS Tiny, white, four-petaled in groups of two to five in forks of stems. Flowers in spring.

FRUIT/SEED Kidney-shaped, covered with hooked bristles, growing on straight stalks.

USES

EDIBLE/OTHER Despite its appearance this herb makes a good vegetable. Cook the young leaves and stems, roast and grind the small seeds to make a coffee substitute. Takes a lot of time to collect the tiny seeds but the coffee is surprisingly good. Roots will dye red. I make a cream with this herb for fading freckles and other blemishes.

MEDICINAL Valuable plant for the lymphatic system. Useful for swollen glands including tonsillitis and adenoid trouble. Widely used for skin conditions, especially dry varieties like psoriasis. Used for kidney ailments of all types. Take internally for ulcers and tumors as it drains the lymph glands. Good antioxidant and general cleanser (alterative). Some authors claim that it is good for losing weight. I use this herb in my tonic tea and preserve it to use for problems with the kidneys and lymph system.

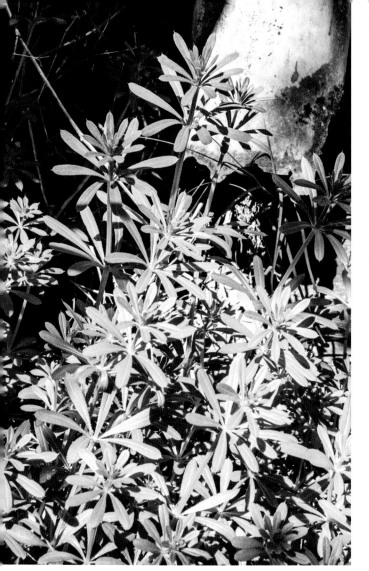
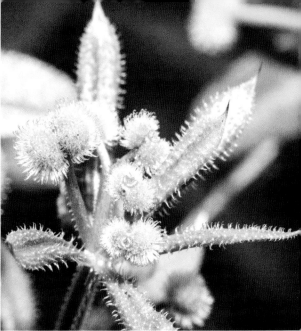
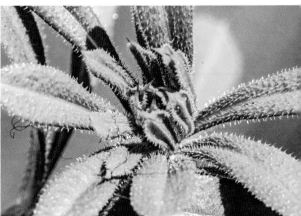

FARM/ENVIR. Stock will eat this herb only when it is young and geese are especially fond of it. This weed grows in crops and contaminates produce and fodder. Invades conservation areas, protected habitats, and causes a serious threat. Along with other weeds dominates the ground layer preventing tree seedlings from growing. Gardeners dislike the messy herb trailing up their fences and trees but it is easy to collect because it mats together. Good for the compost. Indicates soil low in calcium and phosphate and high in potassium and magnesium. Low humus and bacteria with high moisture, hardpan and poor drainage.[8]

FURTHER READING Evaluation of diverse antioxidant activities of *Galium aparine*.[43] *Galium Aparine* as a remedy for chronic ulcers.[44]

WARNING Wear gloves, long sleeves and pants when collecting as small bristles irritate the skin.

CLOVER

White Clover, Dutch Clover

Trifolium repens

DISTRIBUTION Originally from Eurasia and grows worldwide. Common in southern and eastern Australia.

HABITAT This clover has escaped cultivation and now grows prolifically in moist areas being a common weed of lawns, pastures, parks, waste sites, woodlands, roadsides and alpine areas.

DESCRIPTION

Creeping perennial or annual plant in the legume family. Hairless with creeping stems which root at nodes. Abundant in winter and spring.

LEAF Compound leaves have three leaflets, often with distinctive paler V-shaped markings.

FLOWER Known for its fragrant, globular flowers of white with an occasional pinkish tinge on stems 10–20 cm (4–8 in) tall. Mainly flowers in spring.

FRUIT/SEED Tiny pods remain hidden inside old flower parts containing three or four seeds.

USES

EDIBLE/OTHER All clovers are edible. Often known as survival food as you can eat flowers, leaves, stems and root. You can eat them raw or cooked and flower pods can be ground down to a powder. However, there are tastier greens and you will find the white flowers the most edible part; I often put them into salads or make a pleasant tea.

MEDICINAL Infusion of whole plant for rheumatism, tonic, fevers, asthma, colds, coughs and fevers. Infusion of the flowers as an eyewash. American Indians used the plant as a blood cleanser, for boils, sores and wounds. An ointment was made for gout.

FARM/ENVIR. Minor environmental weed that displaces natural vegetation in areas such as

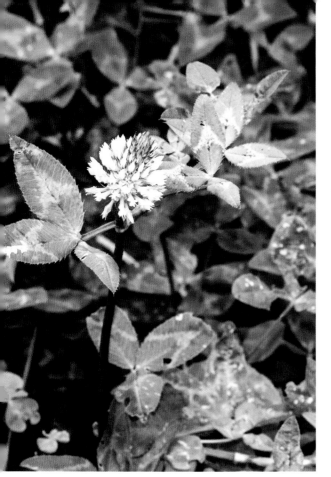
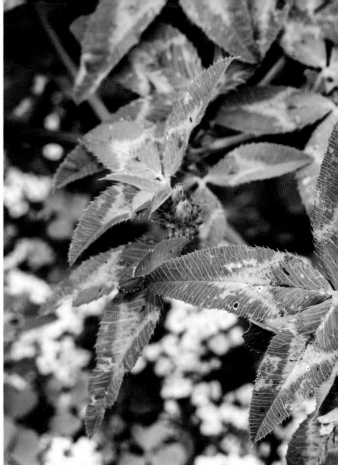

the alpine region. People also dislike them in their lawn as they attract bees. Economically very important in the dairy, meat and wool industries. A pasture with greater than 25% White Clover will result in a manifold increase in stocking rates. It improves soils by fixing atmospheric nitrogen in root nodules. Clover will not grow in acidic soil or soil depleted of potassium. Subterranean Clover being more vigorous will displace White Clover in many situations. Indicates soil high in magnesium, iron, sodium, copper and other minerals. Good drainage.[8]

MAY BE CONFUSED WITH Many other clovers including Red Clover (*T. pratense*). This clover has a pinkish red flower and used for medicinal purposes. Subterranean Clover (*T. subterranean*) which is self-fertilizing and has flowers located beneath the leaves. There are many hybrid clovers so ensure you have the correct seed if planting for medicinal purposes.

FURTHER READING Anticestodal activity of *Trifolium repens*.[45]

WARNING May cause bloat in cattle, goiter in sheep, nutritional myopathy, poor selenium metabolism and cyanide poisoning (low risk). Worry about estrogenic activity but most cultivars of clover usually have a low risk.[46]

COBBLER'S PEGS

Beggar's Tick, Farmer's Friend

Bidens pilosa

DISTRIBUTION Native to South America and now widespread in tropical and temperate climates. Naturalized throughout Australia.

HABITAT Prominent weed of gardens, forests, disturbed areas, roadsides, wastelands and will grow on barren lands.

DESCRIPTION

Erect, annual, hairless or slightly hairy herb up to 2 m (6 ft 6 in) high, growing in the warmer months.

LEAVES Dark green, opposite leaves in groups of three to five, smooth with toothed margins.

FLOWERS Numerous small flower heads, yellow with a ray of white florets.

FRUIT/SEED Clusters of dark seeds have two to three spines at their summit. Barbed projections catch in clothes and animals fur.

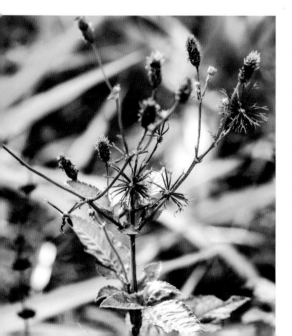

USES

EDIBLE/OTHER Eat young leaves and shoots dried or fresh in sauces and teas. I think there are much nicer wild greens for eating. I prefer to use it as a medicine. In Africa the United Nations Food and Agriculture Organization promoted cultivation as easy to grow, palatable and safe plus nutritious (high in calcium and carotene). Also eaten in Mexico. Tea made from the leaves enjoyed in China and by Texan Indians. Wine made from fermented flowers or leaves in the Philippines.

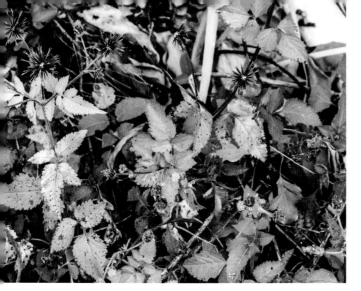
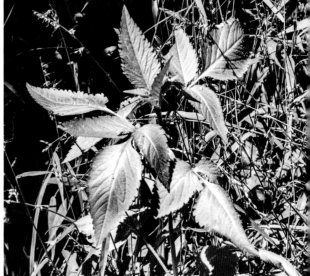

MEDICINAL There have been 116 publications documenting the medicinal use of this plant. In folk medicine it covers 40 categories of illness. Used as a dry powder, decoction, maceration and tincture. Linking traditional usage with rigorous evidence-based scientific study has revealed that this plant has an extraordinary source of phytochemicals that show promise for antitumor, anti-inflammatory, anti-diabetic, antihyperglycemic, antioxidant, immunomodulatory, antimalarial, antibacterial, antifungal, antihypertensive, vasodilatory, antiulcerative and antifungal.[47] Research ongoing.

FARM/ENVIR. Serious weed in many cropping systems where it reduces yield because of its fast growth and competitive abilities, which include allelopathic properties. Also a host for nematodes and viruses. Dense stands will reduce access to roads and trails. Burrs stick into animals' fur and people's clothes and are much disliked. Contaminates grain. This plant seeds prolifically (3,000–6,000 seeds/plant) with seeds highly viable. General tillage can spread the weed. Control with mowing, pulling or extensive cultivation. Stock will eat it when young, toxic in large amounts. This plant grows on our property but Farmer's Friend is more widespread. Indicates soil very low in calcium, phosphate and high in potassium, magnesium and manganese.[8]

MAY BE CONFUSED WITH Other *Bidens* species (four occurring in NSW) all edible with some medicinal use. Farmer's Friend (*B. subalternans*), which has yellow flowers and rays and lower leaves always divided into leaflets. Spanish needles (*B. bipinnata*) with yellow/white rays and yellow center and up to four pairs of toothed leaflets. Bur Marigold (*B. tripartita*) which has a small daisy with a few small yellow rays or none at all and leaves divided into three segments. All have medicinal use.

FURTHER READING *Bidens pilosa* L. (Asteraceae): botanical properties, traditional uses, phytochemistry, and pharmacology.[47] Antimalarial activity of extracts and fractions from *Bidens pilosa* and other *Bidens* species (Asteraceae) correlated with the presence of acetylene and flavonoid compounds.[48]

DANDELION

Wet the Bed, Lion's Tooth

Taraxacum officinale

DISTRIBUTION Native to Eurasia and now widely established. Naturalized in south-east Australia.

HABITAT Found in gardens, parks, wasteland and cultivation. A weed of civilization, following mankind.

DESCRIPTION

Robust perennial herb with long, fleshy taproot containing latex.

LEAVES Long, jagged, hairless leaves rising directly from the root to form a rosette lying close to the ground.

FLOWERS Hollow, leafless flower stalks rise from the root with a single, yellow flower head. Matures to a gossamer ball.

FRUIT/SEED Small seeds fly off with 'parachutes' from the gossamer ball mainly in spring.

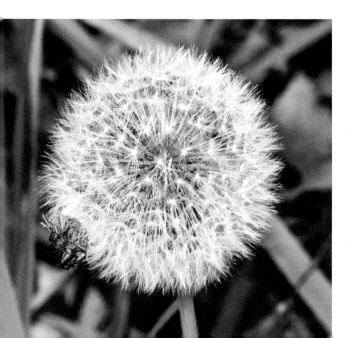

USES

EDIBLE/OTHER Storehouse of minerals, vitamins and enzymes, especially vitamin A and potassium. Pick the leaves before flowering and eat in salads, juice, or cook like spinach. Popular in Italy, France and Greece although, sadly, many societies treat this miraculous plant as a pest. Try tossing leaves with lettuce and tomatoes and homemade dressing or sautéed with olive oil and lemon as

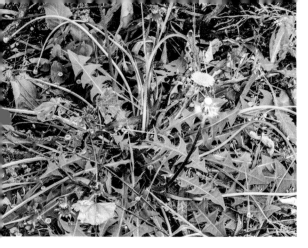

served in Greece. Eat ten stalks every spring and autumn as a tonic. I pick armfuls of the flowers to make a wonderful syrup and use leaves in my tonic tea. Roots are roasted and used as coffee alternative.

MEDICINAL Renowned herb for kidneys and liver. A tea made of the leaves is a safe diuretic (gets rid of fluid), unlike diuretic medication it is high in potassium. Use the roots to treat liver and gall problems, especially jaundice and gallstones. Mild laxative and being a bitter is good for digestion, rheumatism and chronic skin disorders. Also for constipation, anorexia, flatulence and known for its antioxidant, anti-inflammatory, antiheartburn and anticarcinogenic properties. I use this herb a lot in my practice for kidney and liver problems as extracts, tinctures, teas, powders and capsules. Use the white sap on warts and corns.

FARM/ENVIR. Useful plant even for the beekeeper as flowers are high in nectar and pollen. Animals generally graze on dandelions, and it's known to increase the milk production of cows. Birds love the seeds and it is rabbits' favorite food. Wherever you see Dandelion growing it means the soil is good enough to grow legumes like Clover and Lucerne. Earthworms love this plant as its root ventilates the soil and helps produce good humus. Growing these plants will heal and improve poor soils. Powdered roots used for animals as a diuretic. Indicates a soil very low in calcium and very high in potassium, chloride and low in humus with good drainage.[8]

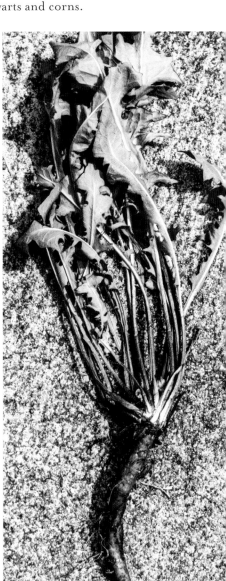

MAY BE CONFUSED WITH False Dandelion (*Hypochoeris species*) which has a branching flower stalk.

FURTHER READING The diuretic effect in human subjects of an extract of *Taraxacum officinale* folium over a single day.[49] Anti-inflammatory effect of *Taraxacum officinale* leaves on lipopolysaccharide-induced inflammatory responses in RAW 264.7 cells.[50] Hypolipidemic and anti-oxidant effects of Dandelion (*Taraxacum officinale*) root and leaf on cholesterol-fed rabbits.[51] Dandelion extracts protect human skin fibroblasts from UVB damage and cellular senescence.[52]

ELDERBERRY

Black Elder

Sambucus nigra

DISTRIBUTION Native to Europe, North Africa and western Asia and now growing worldwide. Naturalized in Australia in higher rainfall areas of New South Wales, Victoria and Tasmania.

HABITAT Growing in hedgerows, along railway embankments, beside rivers, in disturbed areas, woodlands and waste ground. I saw trees in the United Kingdom but was surprised to see them in Vietnam around the villages.

DESCRIPTION

Short-lived, scruffy, woody shrub 1–6 m (3 ft 3 in–19 ft 7 in) high.

LEAVES Opposite leaflets with toothed margins on leaf blade.

FLOWERS Distinctive, white, dome-like, masses of flowers growing terminally. They have a light perfume and flower mostly in the warmer months.

FRUIT/SEED Bunches of drooping purplish-black small berries each containing four to five seeds.

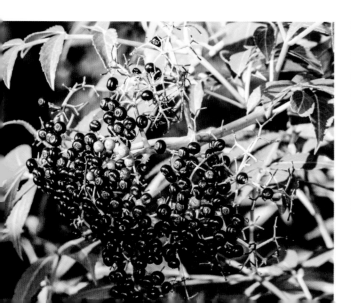

USES

EDIBLE/OTHER Revered for centuries, now this plant has become very commercial with orchards grown for the flowers and berries. A wide range of cordials and wines are sold and have become so popular one firm in the United Kingdom employs 600 people in season to pick the flowers from the hedgerows to make products. Avoid

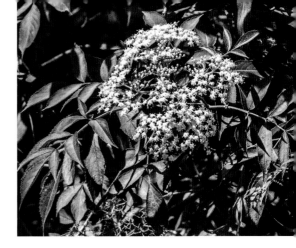

eating raw flowers and fruit as they contain an alkaloid; this can be neutralized by heating. Makes excellent jams, fritters, pies and other baked goods. In season, I make elder fritters and the cordial – delicious! Ripe berries used to color wines. Dyes, perfumes, wooden products especially musical instruments are made from this tree. I make a very popular Rose and Elder moisturizing cream and lotion, which is good for normal skin. There is also much folklore attached to this tree.

MEDICINAL To extol its virtues would take pages in fact in 1644 a 230-page book was written on the virtues of Elder covering everything from toothache to plague. It is a veritable medicine chest by itself. So many uses. Leaves primarily for bruises, sprains, wounds and chilblains. Flowers for respiratory problems such as colds, flu, (extracts showing inhibition to 11 strains of influenza virus), asthma, chronic bronchitis, hayfever and sinus. It is specific for catarrhal deafness. Berries also have many uses including rheumatism. Other popular uses are for fevers, pleurisy, measles, laryngitis and any head congestion, boils, inflamed eyes, digestive troubles, inflammation, skin problems and as an antioxidant. Bark used as a strong purgative. Administer this herb by giving capsules, tablets, extracts, teas, syrups and lozenges. I make a popular Winter blend tea containing Elder and other herbs. New research also shows promise for diabetes.

FARM/ENVIR. Rapidly colonizes disturbed areas and displaces native species. Needs good rainfall. I have lost many Elders due to lack of moisture. Does make a good hedge but can become scraggly if not maintained. It is toxic to stock, however I always lose half my Elders if they are hanging over the fence as my goats love them, cattle and sheep will eat them as well. In small amounts toxicity does not seem to be an issue. If sheep eat the bark and young shoots, it will cure foot rot. The birds love the berries, but they are not so good for chickens.

MAY BE CONFUSED WITH American Elder (*Sambucus nigra* L. ssp. *canadensis*) is a native to America and botanically very close to Black Elder. A great deal of research has been carried out on this plant and it has similar medicinal values to Black Elder. Many species are widely cultivated for their ornamental leaves, flowers and fruit.

FURTHER READING Elderberry as a medicinal plant.[53] Elderberry (*Sambucus nigra* L.) wine: a product rich in health promoting compounds.[54] Gastrointestinal digested *Sambucus nigra* L. fruit extract protects in vitro cultured human colon cells against oxidative stress.[55]

WARNING Flowers, fruit and leaves contain a strong alkaloid.

ENGLISH DAISY

Bellis perennis

DISTRIBUTION Native to the Mediterranean region and now widespread. Growing in cooler areas of Australia, especially Victoria and Tasmania.

HABITAT Garden escapee now growing in lawns, recreation areas, vacant blocks, stream banks, sand dunes, grasslands and wasteland.

DESCRIPTION

Perennial, low-growing plant with creeping rhizomes that create a mat.

LEAVES Small, oval, green leaves that start with a rosette.

FLOWERS Small, daisy-like flower with yellow centers and white petals, occasionally with a pink tinge, growing singularly on leafless stalks. Flowers in spring and early summer. Longer in cooler areas.

FRUIT/SEED Small, brown and shaped like an almond.

USES

EDIBLE Leaves and flowers eaten raw or cooked. Has a slight acrid flavor but I enjoy having the little flowers as a decoration in my vegetable and fruit salads.

MEDICINAL Traditionally an ointment is made from the leaves for wounds, bruises, eczema and other skin conditions. Used as a tonic and appetizer; for flu and colds, for digestive problems including liver disorders; anti-inflammatory so good for joint pains and arthritis; helps with heavy menstruation; mouth ulcers and even for breast cancer and HIV support.

FARM/ENVIR. Environmental weed in cooler areas, growing as a mat so that natives cannot propagate. Problem in conservation and natural reserves. This plant does not grow as a weed in my area. I plant these delightful little flowers but when it gets very hot in summer,

they tend to die off. At my sister's place in Tasmania, they come up all over her lawn.

FURTHER READING The evaluation of topical administration of *Bellis perennis* fraction on circular excision wound healing in Wistar albino rats.[56] Effects of common daisy (*Bellis perennis* L.) aqueous extracts on anxiety-like behavior and spatial memory performance in Wistar albino rats.[57]

FALSE DANDELION

Flatweed, Common Catsear

Hypochoeris radicata

DISTRIBUTION Native of Eurasia and North Africa spread into Americas, Japan, Australia and New Zealand. Most widespread weed in south-eastern Australia.

HABITAT Found in lawns, gardens, roadsides, pastures, abandoned cultivation, disturbed wasteland and sand banks.

DESCRIPTION

Perennial herb 15–80 cm (6–31 in) with deep taproot.

LEAVES A flat, basal rosette of club-shaped, variable leaves with rounded tip. Covered in fine hairs.

FLOWERS Bright yellow daisy flowers growing on leafless flower stalks that branch and have two to seven terminal flowers. Flowering throughout the year with a flush in spring and early summer.

FRUIT/SEED Flower matures into a small gossamer ball that releases single small seeds on 'parachutes' into the wind.

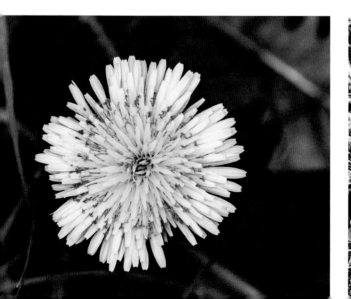
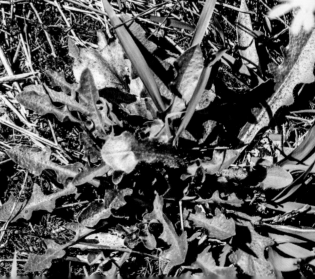

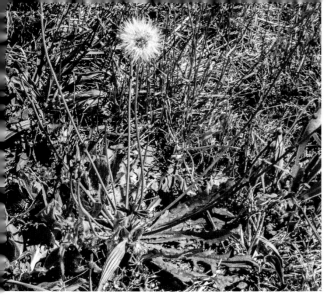
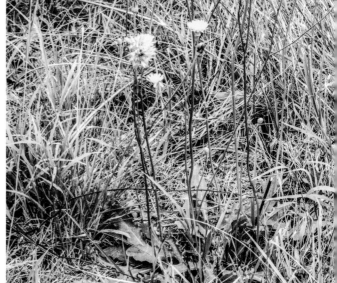

USES

EDIBLE/OTHER Young leaves are a good green to eat being mild and tender. Good in pies, quiches, soups and salads. In nineteenth century Europe, it was a popular pot herb and grown in gardens for the table. The roasted roots make a coffee substitute. This herb grows in large numbers on our property and I enjoy eating the flowers.

MEDICINAL In Nilgiri, India this herb is popular with the traditional healers for treating inflammation, infectious diseases, cancer, wound healing and skin diseases. Root extract gives the best results for infections.[59] Other uses are as an antioxidant, antimicrobial, protects liver and helps with kidney problems. High in vitamin C.

FARMING/ENVIR. False dandelions smother the ground around them and do not allow grasses to grow and limit grazing. Aerate the soil and apply humus and nutrients and these plants will diminish. They have deep roots, which allow them to be drought resistant and survive even on sandy, poor soils. Not toxic to livestock however if horses eat excessive amounts they may develop stringhalt. Good honey plant. Indicates soil low in calcium and very low in potassium with low humus and bacteria.[8]

MAY BE CONFUSED WITH Smooth Catsears (*H. glabra*) which has few or no hairs on the leaves and unlike False Dandelion their seeds have no beaks. However, these two plants have created hybrids and it often makes it difficult to identify between species. Dandelion (*Taraxacum officinale*) has singular hollow stems with one flower on each.

FURTHER READING Phytochemical analysis and evaluation of leaf and root parts of the medicinal herb, *Hypochaeris radicata* L. for in vitro antioxidant activities.[58] In vitro antibacterial activity of leaf and root extracts of *Hypochaeris radicata* L. (Asteraceae) – a medicinal plant species inhabiting the high hills of Nilgiri, the western ghats.[59]

WARNING Avoid horses grazing on large amounts of this plant as it can cause stringhalt.

FAT HEN

White Goosefoot, Lamb's Quarter

Chenopodium album

DISTRIBUTION Cosmopolitan. Naturalized in temperate and subtropical regions of Australia.

HABITAT Found in the garden, summer crops, disturbed sites, river banks, roadsides, bushland and wasteland.

DESCRIPTION

Non-aromatic, erect, annual herb 20 cm to 1.5 m (8 in to 4 ft 9 in), much branched, growing in the warmer months.

LEAVES Oval toothed, dull green upper, mealy white beneath.

FLOWERS Dense green, mealy spikes, reddish-brown as it matures.

FRUIT/SEED Dark, round and small, ripe late summer.

USES

EDIBLE/OTHER Excellent worldwide herb, used for thousands of years, (found in remains of ancient Tollund Man) and high in nutrients. Seeds eaten raw, toasted or ground into flour to make bread. I regularly use the leaves in salads, rissoles, quiche or casserole. Related to Quinoa.

MEDICINAL Important Ayurvedic medicinal plant with pharmacological studies proving its use in sugar imbalances, anti-bacterial and anti-inflammatory problems; helping the liver and relieving spasms. Used elsewhere as a tonic, for digestive ailments, parasites, laxative, eye diseases, throat problems and digestive problems. Poultice used externally for skin sores and burns.

FARM/ENVIR. It is one of the world's most widespread weeds with seeds viable for 30 to 40 years. Agricultural and environmental weed invading natural vegetation and conservation

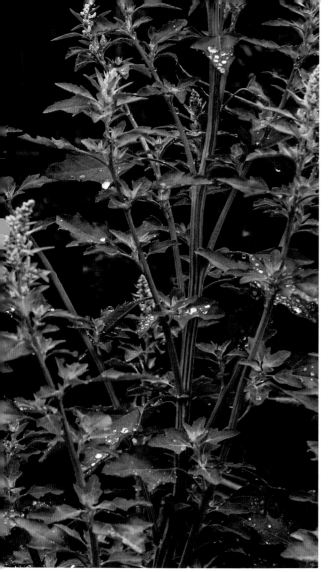
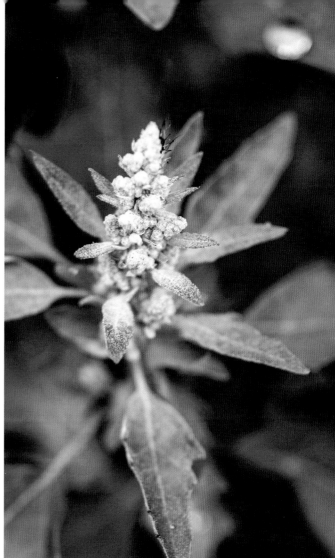

areas. In Canada grown for sheep and pigs, elsewhere for birds and poultry. I give the leaves to my chooks and I get lovely yellow yolks. Leaf paste on wounds and sores of cattle. Its presence can indicate soil low in phosphate and high in potassium and sulfate.[8]

MAY BE CONFUSED WITH Mexican Tea (*C. ambrosioides*) All aerial parts have an ant-like odor. Good King Henry (*C. bonus-henricus*) which looks like *C.* Fat Hen except it has a fleshier stem, which is hollow. Native Fish Weed (*Einadia trigonos*) a trailing herb with slender stems. All plants edible.

FURTHER READING Anthelmintic activity against trichostrongylid nematodes of sheep.[60] Use as an anti-breast cancer bioagent.[61]

WARNING Contains oxalates.

FENNEL

Wild Fennel, Aniseed

Foeniculum vulgare

DISTRIBUTION Native to the Mediterranean region and now cosmopolitan worldwide. In Australia, grows mainly in the coastal and sub coastal, southern and south-east regions.

HABITAT Weed of wasteland, alluvial flats, riverbanks, roadsides, grasslands and irrigation ditches.

DESCRIPTION

Strongly aromatic, long-lived perennial with an aniseed flavor. Stout with numerous stems 1.5–3 m (4 ft 9 in–9 ft 8 in) in height with a strong taproot.

LEAVES Finely divided, lacy, thread-like.

FLOWERS Umbrella-like groups of numerous small, yellow flowers at ends of branches. Flowers in summer.

FRUIT/SEED Green changing to grey-brown when ripe in summer/autumn.

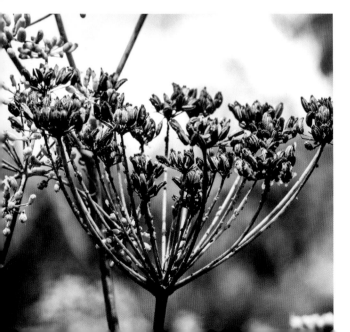

USES

EDIBLE/OTHER Leaves, swollen stems, roots, green or ripe seeds eaten fresh or cooked in dishes. Anglo-Saxon recipes used a lot of Fennel and its culinary use is thought to have come from Italy – 'helpeth to digest the crude qualitie of fish and other viscous meats'. (John Parkinson, *Theatrum Botanicum*, 1640) I have a lot of wild Fennel and love eating the fresh green seeds.

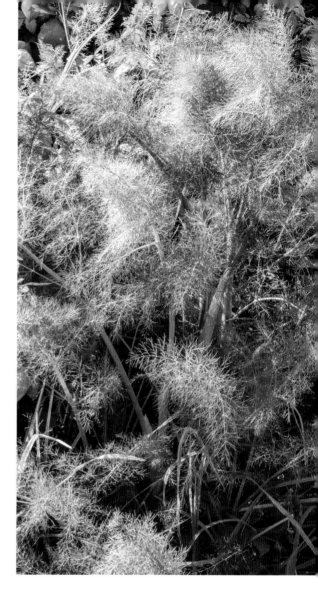

MEDICINAL Good for griping and intestinal colic. I have good results making a colic mix for babies using fennel, aniseed and dill seeds with chamomile. Cook in soups and stews to ease flatulence. Good for mother's milk, bringing up phlegm, and calming the gut. Ayurvedic medicine uses the dry leaves to make a tea to treat coughs, excess fluid, diarrhea, pain and parasites. Also as an anti-microbial agent, antioxidant, insecticide and to reduce blood pressure. Seeds chewed to abate hunger and help with digestion. I make a successful cream using the essential oil for getting rid of excess hair in women.

FARM Significant and widespread environmental weed as it out-competes small, native understory shrubs and ground cover. Minor problem in pastures as animals graze on it. Cattle and goats will increase their milk supply but it does taint milk. Grow away from other vegetables and herbs as it makes a poor companion. Deep roots can be a problem but over the years, I have found that covering in carpet will deter its growth. Its presence can indicate low calcium and phosphate in the soil, poor humus, low moisture and compacted soil.[8]

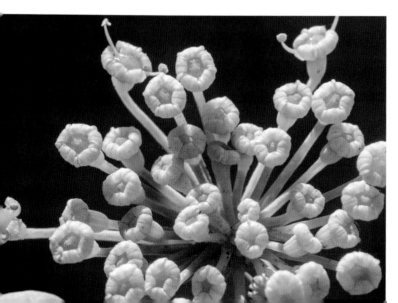

FURTHER READING Clinical trials showed good results in IBS, colitis, cough, sleeping, infantile colic, dysmenorrhea (latter two using Fennel essential oil). A cream using 1–2% extract reduced hair growth (hirsutism).[62]

WARNING Avoid if you have an allergy to the Umbelliferae family (carrots, celery).

FEVERFEW

Featherfew, Febrifuge plant

Chrysanthemum parthenium/Tanacetum parthenium L.

DISTRIBUTION Native of south-east Europe now widespread. Naturalized in south-east Australia.

HABITAT Grown as an ornamental and now a garden escapee growing outside its native range. It has become an invasive weed in gardens, wasteland, wayside and mountain shrub.

DESCRIPTION

Perennial, sometimes biennial about 90 cm (3 ft) tall, with many branched stems. Initially soft but becoming woody.

LEAF Light green, feathery and strongly scented.

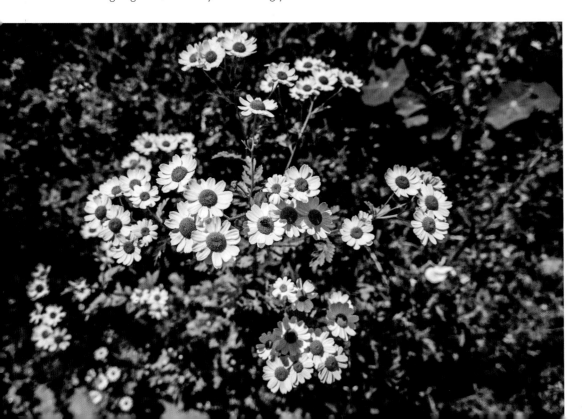

FLOWER Numerous flower heads like small daisies with yellow centers and white petals. Flowering spring and summer.

FRUIT/SEED Small numerous seeds.

USES

EDIBLE/OTHER Bitter tasting but occasionally used in cooking to 'cut' the grease.

MEDICINAL Main use is for migraines. Best to take daily as a preventative. Fresh herb gives you the best results. Also used for arthritis as a good anti-inflammatory. Helps as a mild sedative for hysteria, headaches, fever, labor, menstruation, nervous problems, pain, tinnitus and vertigo. Externally use fresh leaf for insect bites and useful for inflammatory skin complaints (use the tea). Active ingredient parthenolide is showing promise in cancer research. Sold as tea, extract, capsules and tablets.

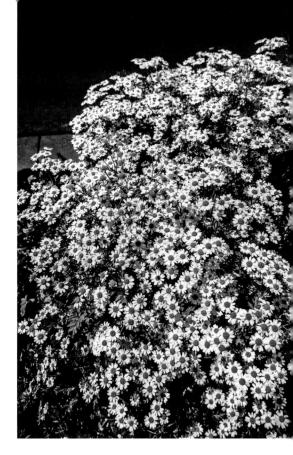

FARM/ENVIR. Many people grow this ornamental daisy in their garden without knowing its medicinal uses. Now there is a double flowered variety, which is not medicinal. I grow numerous plants so that I can have a good supply of dried flowers for the capsules we make to sell at our clinic, mainly for migraines and headaches. Minor weed, stock will usually avoid it. Good insecticide, use as an alternative to pyrethrum. Early American settlers grew this herb as a border around their vegetable gardens to protect their produce against insects. There is a small amount of commercial growing of this plant.

MAY BE CONFUSED WITH Chamomile (*Matricaria recutita*) which has similar flowers but a finer, feathery leaf. The center of the flower is more conical.

FURTHER READING The efficacy and safety of Feverfew (*Tanacetum parthenium* L.).[63] Anti-microbial properties and possible role in host-pathogen interactions of parthenolide.[64] Feverfew (*Tanacetum parthenium* L.): A systematic review.[65]

WARNING Side effects are usually minor such as mouth ulcers. Avoid during pregnancy. Do not take internally if you develop a rash on contact with the plant. If you are hypersensitive to members of the daisy family avoid this plant. You may suffer withdrawal symptoms if you have been taking the herb for some time – you may get rebound headaches, muscle and joint pains.

FISHBONE FERN

Common Sword Fern

Nephrolepis cordifolia

DISTRIBUTION Native of northern Australia and naturalized in tropical and subtropical regions of the world including New Zealand, parts of America and the Pacific Islands.

HABITAT Found in natural forests, scrub, coastland, urban areas, disturbed sites and wetlands.

DESCRIPTION

Semi-evergreen fern with underground stems that form dense clumps. Distinctive round tubers are found on these rhizomes.

LEAVES First appearing as slender wiry 'fiddleheads' and growing into upright, drooping fronds up to 50 cm-1 m (1 ft 6 in–3 ft 3 in) long. Leaves divided into numerous alternative arranged arrow 'leaflets'.

FRUIT/SEED Older leaves have spores on the underside. Spreads by rhizomes or by windblown spores.

USES

EDIBLE/OTHER The watery root tubers are cooked and eaten. The fiddleheads are also edible. Soak and cook before eating.

MEDICINAL Use the fresh fronds in a tea to drink for coughs and amnesia. Rhizomes are cooling, antibacterial and chewed for nose blockage. Eaten to relieve chest congestion, indigestion, fever and to help liver and kidneys. Rhizome paste relieves body ache, scabies and headache. Root juice for a cough and colds.

FARM/ENVIR. Ornamental plant, which has escaped from cultivation into natural areas and is now an environmental weed. Has an aggressive growing habit forming dense stands that exclude native species. Easy to dig up the clumping mats in the early stages as roots are not deep. In New Zealand it is illegal to sell or cultivate the plant and it is known as an invasive species in Florida. Research showed screening for heavy metal tolerance in common Australian fern species; showed that this fern can absorb a wide range of heavy metals and may be used to revitalize contaminated soils.[66]

MAY BE CONFUSED WITH Other native ferns such as Rasp Fern (*Doodia aspera*) with its slightly serrated harsh fronds and Sickle Fern (*Pellaea falcate*) which has distinctive black, wiry stems.

FURTHER READING Heavy metal tolerance in common fern species.[66] In vitro anti-bacterial and anti-fungal properties of aqueous and non-aqueous frond extracts of *Psilotum nudum*, *Nephrolepis biserrata* and *Nephrolepis cordifolia*.[67]

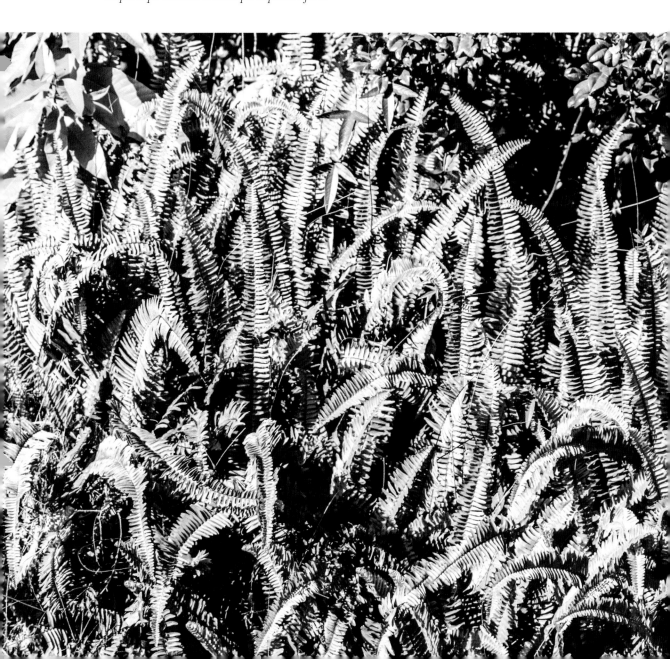

FLEABANE

Flaxleaf Fleabane

Conyza bonariensis

DISTRIBUTION Native to North America and now growing worldwide. Naturalized throughout Australia, especially the south east.

HABITAT Widespread weed growing in wasteland, old fields, irrigation areas, roadsides and paddocks. Seasonally abundant.

DESCRIPTION

Erect, hairy, annual herb up to 20–75 cm (8–30 in) high, woody at base and extensively branched with outside stems taller than central stem. Grows spring to autumn.

LEAF Crowded, ascending, narrow, grey-green leaves undulating at margins with a basal leaf rosette. Leaves are slightly hairy.

FLOWERS Numerous buds mature to form whitish colored small gossamer balls, attached to seeds. Specialized leaf holding the flower heads (bracts) tipped with a few long hairs.

FRUIT/SEED The tiny seeds are dispersed by wind on their tiny 'parachutes'. Each plant produces about 3,000 seeds and research shows they can travel up to 100 km (62 mi).

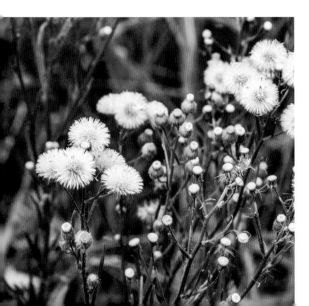

USES

EDIBLE/OTHER Not used for culinary purposes. These plants are burnt to drive away fleas and insects. Use an infusion of this herb or any other plants of the *Conyza* species in your dog's next bath along with other strong smelling herbs to treat problems with fleas. I have told many students and clients to do this when their dog has a bad itch from fleas and have obtained good results.

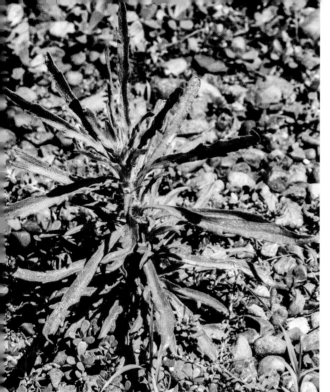
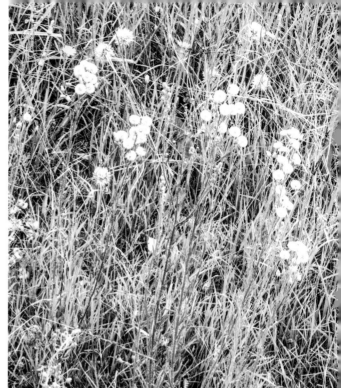

MEDICINAL Whole plant for intestinal troubles, diarrhea, dysentery, rheumatism, ringworm and sore throat. Flowering branches are good for fluid problems. Crushed stems and leaves used to make a poultice to draw infection from wounds. Roots are for stomach problems.[68]

FARM/ENVIR. Five plants in the *Conyza* species grow in Australia. The species is rated as herbicide-resistant weeds due to their ability to reproduce quickly and to disperse seed widely. Occasionally can be a problem with cultivation which is controlled by tillage and planting a stronger cover crop. This plant spreads across non-cropping areas and is difficult to control. Generally not grazed by livestock. Use the herb for cuts, wounds and mosquito bites on your animals. Also used as a fish poison. Indicates soil very low in calcium, phosphate and very high in potassium, magnesium and zinc. Poor humus and bacteria and low moisture.[8]

MAY BE CONFUSED WITH Four other species similar in appearance and often growing together. Canadian Fleabane (*C. canadensis*) grows up to 1.5 m (4 ft 9 in) high and bracts have a brownish inner surface and pappus cream; Tall Fleabane (*C. albida*) grows about 1 m (3 ft 3 in) high with one central stem and no long hairs near the apex of bracts; two other species previously included under *C. canadensis* are *C. bilbaoana* and *C. parva*.

FURTHER READING Antioxidant and antibacterial activities of extracts from *Conyza bonariensis* growing in Yemen.[69] Gut modulator effects of *Conyza bonariensis* explain its traditional use in constipation and diarrhea.[70]

FOUR O'CLOCK

Marvel of Peru, Clavillia

Mirabilis jalapa

DISTRIBUTION Native of tropical America now naturalized in many tropical and subtropical regions including, in Australia, the central and north coast of New South Wales, as well as Queensland and Victoria.

HABITAT Grown as a garden ornamental that has escaped cultivation and now grows in neglected gardens, crops, wasteland and other disturbed areas, especially near habitation.

DESCRIPTION

An erect, rather scraggly, long-lived perennial up to 3 m (9 ft 8 in) in height. A prolific grower in the warmer months. Frost tender.

LEAVES Oval and smooth.

FLOWERS Colors range from white, pink, yellow and a mixture of these colors. Flowers are funnel-shaped opening in late afternoon or in cloudy weather with a beautiful perfume.

FRUIT/SEED Round, rough, black seeds with a brown seed inside.

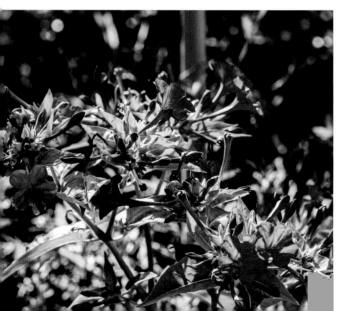
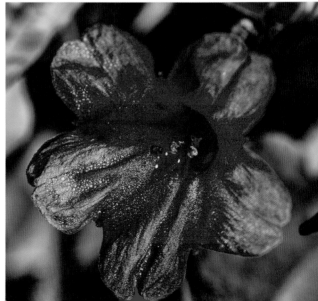

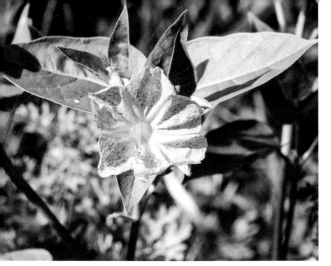
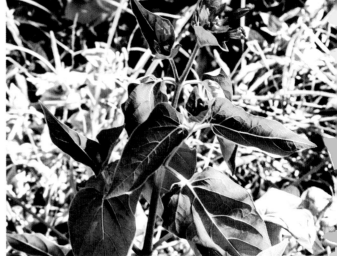

USES

EDIBLE/OTHER Leaves are not pleasant to eat and only eat small amounts cooked, do not eat raw. Cooked with pork as a tonic. Flowers used as a dye for coloring cakes and jellies. I planted these flowers in my garden 30 years ago and I'm now rewarded with lovely scraggly plants and an abundance of perfumed flowers opening about 4 o'clock. Many little seedlings appear after the frost, which I cull each spring.

MEDICINAL Traditionally many countries have used the leaves, flowers and root for medicinal purposes. A great deal of information has come from the natives of South America, Mexico and from India. As a broad-spectrum antimicrobial for bacterial, fungal and viral infections; for candida and yeast infections; as a bowel cleanser and laxative and for skin problems (eczema, dermatitis, acne, rashes, liver spots, skin fungi, ringworm) and the root used for parasites. Traditionally decoctions, juices, dried and ground leaves, flowers, and root (used as a paste for external problems) and tea used. Now capsules and extracts are popular.[71]

FARM/ENVIR. Minor environmental weed in many parts of the world. Has the ability to compete with indigenous vegetation. Will withstand droughts due to its large tuberous roots. Invasive in East Africa. Mirabilis antiviral proteins (MAPs) have been isolated from the seeds, leaves and roots and found to be very effective at protecting economically important crops such as tobacco, corn and potatoes against a large variety of plant viruses.[71] The root paste is used on livestock for sunstroke and infectious diseases. Indicates soil very low in calcium, phosphate and very high in potassium and magnesium and other minerals. Low in humus, moisture with good drainage.[8]

FURTHER READING Inhibition of histamine mediated responses by *Mirabilis jalapa*: confirming traditional claims made about antiallergic and antiasthmatic activity.[72] Anti-inflammatory activity of aqueous extract of *Mirabilis jalapa* L. leaves.[73]

WARNING Seeds and roots contain neurotoxic chemicals. Leaves minor toxicity.

FUMITORY

Wall Fumitory, Smoke Weed

Fumaria muralis

DISTRIBUTION Native to Eurasia and spread to temperate regions of the world. Naturalized in southern Australia. There are 50 species of *Fumaria* with eight recorded in Australia.

HABITAT In gardens, cultivated ground, crops and wasteland.

DESCRIPTION

Sprawling, annual, delicate herb with many branches of soft stems to 30 cm (12 in) long. Grows in winter and spring.

LEAVES Deeply dissected, greyish-green leaves growing opposite (carrot-like).

FLOWERS Small, tubular, pink-red flowers with dark tips growing in loose, terminal racemes. Approximately 12 flowers in each inflorescence.

FRUIT/SEED Rounded and on short stalks.

USES

EDIBLE/OTHER Used only for medicinal purposes.

MEDICINAL In tropical Africa this plant is used as a strong decoction in the bath for eczema, acne, ringworm, scurvy itch and wounds. Eye bath for conjunctivitis. Internally as a tonic and stimulant, for bile secretion regulation, liver stimulating, laxative, purgative, antidiabetic and good for cholesterol. Syrup for children with gastroenteritis. I have made an ointment using this herb for dermatitis with good results. European Fumitory (*F. officinalis*) has similar uses but it is the best medicinally.

FARM/ENVIR. Can successfully compete with existing vegetation and in places like the Murrumbidgee catchment in southern New South Wales it has become an increasing problem in annual crops. Tillage will deplete the seed bank. It covers my garden and my orchard in the cooler months but is very easy to pull up and put into the compost.

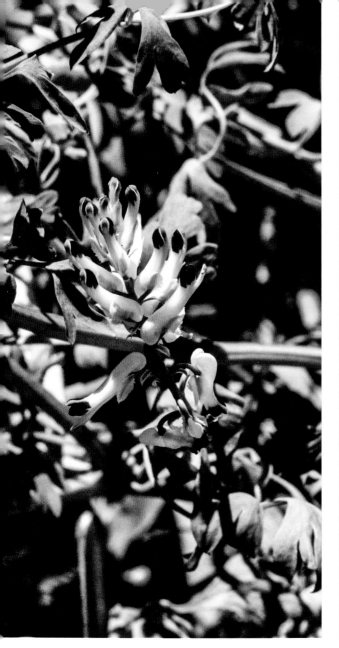
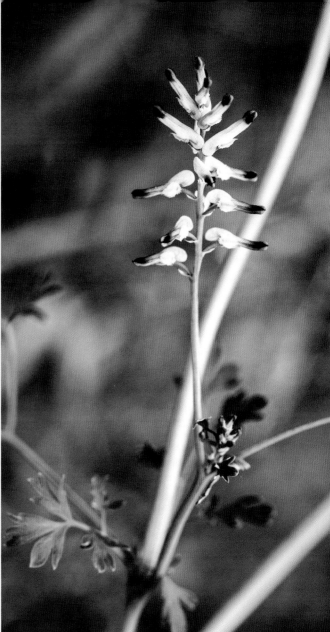

MAY BE CONFUSED WITH European Fumitory (*F. officinalis*) has the same colored flowers but has 20 flowers each flower head and fruit has large shallow pit at its apex. White Flowered Fumitory (*F. capreolata* L.) has white with purple-tipped flowers. Wall Fumitory may hybridize with White Flowered Fumitory.

FURTHER READING Antioxidant and antilipoperoxidant activities of alkaloid and phenolic extracts of eight *Fumaria* species.[74] Plant resources of Tropical Africa.[74a]

WARNING Low toxicity.

GOLDEN ROD

Canadian Golden Rod

Solidago canadensis var. *scabra*

DISTRIBUTION Native to America and Canada and introduced to Europe, parts of Asia, especially China and Australasia. Naturalized in eastern Australia.

HABITAT Commonly found in neglected gardens, poorly managed pastures, abandoned fields, wasteland near habitation, along roads, water courses and on railway embankments. Prefers higher rainfall areas.

DESCRIPTION

Comes from a variable species S. canadensis and has the same qualities. Tall growing, erect, perennial herb up to 1.5 m (4 ft 9 in) in height. Has an underground root system from which new shoots grow. Hairless at the base but hairy stems and leaves above.

LEAVES Narrow, serrated, alternate and attached directly to the stem.

FLOWERS Conspicuous, bright yellow inflorescence in a pyramid shape growing terminally. Flowers in autumn.

FRUIT/SEED Each flower dries to form a pappus with a small seed attached that is dispersed by the wind.

USES

EDIBLE/OTHER Young leaves and flowering stems are cooked. Seed used to thicken soup. Make a tea from flowers and leaves. Used in vinegars and to produce oil and dye.

MEDICINAL Infusion of leaves and flowers as a wash for boils, open sores and skin irritations; treats urinary problems and used as a general anti-inflammatory. The American Indians made tea and mixtures from compounds of flowers and roots to cleanse system, used as a sedative, for diarrhea, fevers and flu. One tribe chewed crushed flowers for sore throat and drank the tea for body pain.[75] This plant is closely related to European Goldenrod

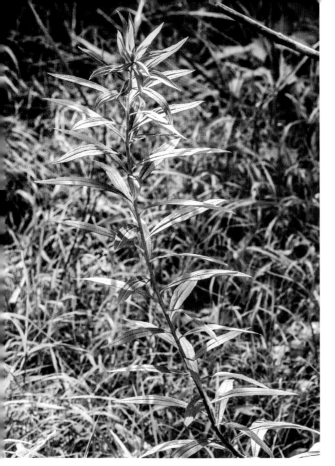 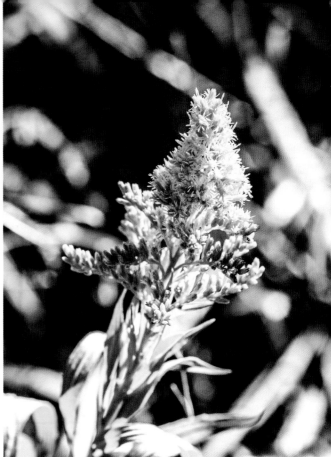

(*S. virgaurea*) which is used for chronic sinusitis, hayfever, serious ear problems, sore throats, catarrhal deafness, influenza and catarrh from nose and throat. Also used for kidney or bladder stones both as treatment and prevention along with rheumatoid and osteoarthritis. I make a Breathe Easy tea and this is one of the main ingredients.

FARM/ENVIR. Its large root system, vigorous growth combined with allelopathic effects leads to gross changes in native vegetation and fauna. Easily controlled by tilling but difficult to control in natural areas. Perennial gardens and forest nurseries also find it a pest. Good for attracting beneficial insects to the garden such as ladybirds, lacewings and hoverflies. Bees love the pollen and nectar. Also a soil stabilizer and source of food and shelter for wildlife. Will tolerate some dry conditions but I have lost mine in droughts when I have forgotten to water it. Fair-to-good forage for cattle, sheep and horses. Indicates soil low in calcium and high in potassium with low humus and high moisture.[8]

MAY BE CONFUSED WITH Tall Goldenrod (*Solidago altissima* subsp. *altissima*) which is very similar to the Canadian Goldenrod whose leaves are more sharply serrated. Shares the same medicinal qualities.

FURTHER READING HPLC investigation of antioxidant components in *Solidago* herbs.[76]

HAWTHORN

May, Whitethorn

Crataegus monogyna/Crataegus laevigata

DISTRIBUTION Native to Europe, North Africa and western Asia and now widespread in countries throughout the world. Naturalized in south-eastern Australia.

HABITAT Considered an understory species in its native habitat. Prefers moist to damp disturbed places such as lake margins, and open forest.

DESCRIPTION

Large deciduous shrub or small tree 4–6 m (13–20 ft) high. Has many spreading, thorny branches.

LEAVES Alternate, variable, triangular or ovate in outline, deeply lobed and toothed at the tip.

FLOWERS Five-petaled white, cream, pink or red flowers cluster along the branches. They have a strong scent. Flower in spring.

FRUIT/SEED Clusters of shiny red berries with yellow flesh. Taste is neutral. *C. monogyna* has one seed/fruit and *C. laevigata* has two or three seeds/fruit.

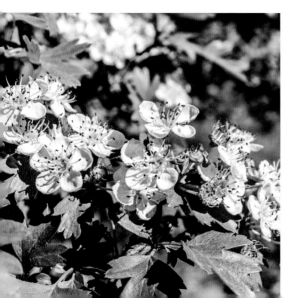

USES

EDIBLE/OTHER In England the fruit and flowers are used in many products. Flowers make a pleasant wine and add color to a salad. The berries make a tasty liqueur, sauce and haw jams and jellies are popular especially as the fruit has a high pectin content. Green shoots are also edible. Berries used in cosmetic and hair care products to increase hydration and elasticity of the skin. Excellent for woodwork and honey.

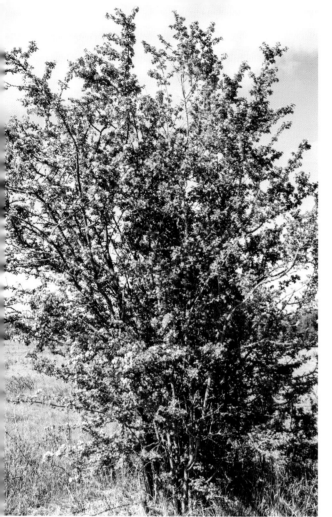
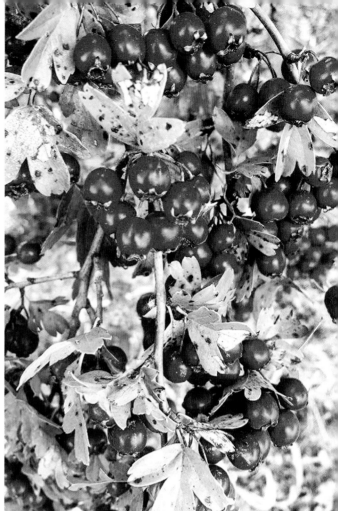

MEDICINAL Renowned as a heart tonic. What would herbalists do without this precious herb! One of the best tonic remedies for the heart and circulatory system, used for mild high blood pressure, for long-term treatment of heart failure and weakness. Hawthorn will move the heart to a normal function in a gentle way. Has antioxidant qualities, helping with mild anxiety, hot flushes and used topically for acne. I sell this herb in teas, extracts and capsules and I am so thankful I have this herb to offer my clients.

FARM/ENVIR. Brought to Australia as a hedge plant it has now become a noxious weed in South Australia and Victoria, as it forms dense thickets that provides home for foxes and rabbits. It is a host for light brown apple moth. Spines deter grazing, however, it does provide excellent stock shelter and in many areas is still grown as an impenetrable hedge. Used to revegetate land, reclamation of wasteland and mine spoils. Relatively tolerant to air pollution, thus good to grow beside motorways.[77]

FURTHER READING Antioxidant activity, liver function test, heart disease, clinical trials in congestive heart failure, blood pressure and acne.[78]

HEARTSEASE

Wild Pansy, Johnny-jump-up

Viola tricolor

DISTRIBUTION Cosmopolitan, growing profusely in Europe and North America. Naturalized in Australia in small pockets mainly in southern New South Wales, Victoria and Tasmania.

HABITAT Prefers a moist fertile soil often near habitation. In other countries grows in hedge banks, waste ground and in cultivation.

DESCRIPTION

Annual or short-lived perennial, somewhat straggly and branched to 25 cm (10 in) tall.

LEAVES Opposite, deeply cut into round lobes, the terminal leaf being considerably larger.

FLOWERS Three-colored petals – white, yellow and purple, or a combination of these colors. Has a long flowering season, a flush in spring.

FRUIT/SEED Little capsules of seeds, which when mature open by three valves.

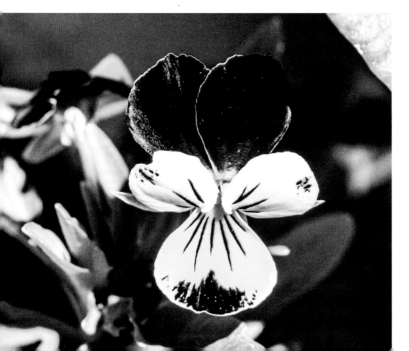

USES

EDIBLE/OTHER Edible flowers used in salads, freeze in ice blocks for drinks and crystallize flowers to decorate cakes. Use leaves and flowers to make a refreshing tea. The leaves also used instead of litmus paper in acid and alkali tests. The plant is steeped in tradition and beliefs.

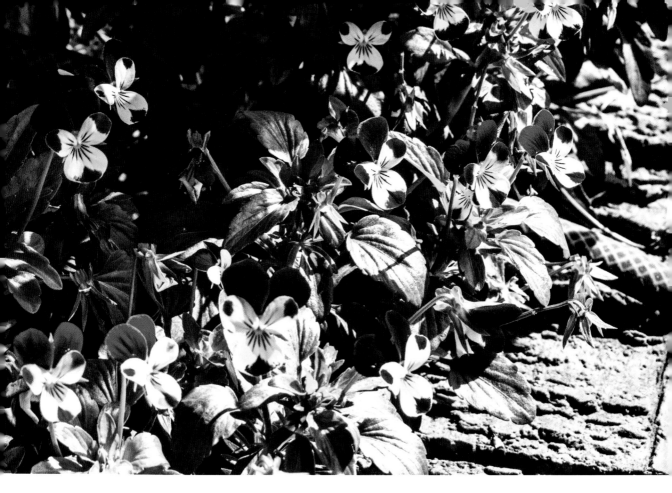

MEDICINAL Once cultivated medicinally and used extensively by herbalists for 'blood purification'. Use for a wide range of skin disorders such as nappy rash, varicose ulcers, skin sores, eczema, cradle cap, weeping sores and insect bites. Make a tea or syrup for coughs and fevers. Helps blood vessels, indigestion, urinary system, inflammation and immune system. Take as tea, tincture or extract, externally as a poultice or cream.

FARM/ENVIR. Not a problem on a broader scale, growing well in sheltered areas where other grasses struggle. Minor problem of cultivated fields. I love growing it in the garden – so colorful and it lasts most of the year in a shady spot.

MAY BE CONFUSED WITH The myriad of garden pansies originated from the wild *V. tricolor*. Sweet violet (*V. odorata*) is also a close relative but its purple flowers are distinctively different.

FURTHER READING The cumulation of Wild Pansy (*Viola tricolor* L.) accessions: the possibility of species preservation and usage in medicine.[79] Immunosuppressive activity of an aqueous *Viola tricolor* herbal extract.[80] Antioxidant and antibacterial activities of extracts from *Conyza bonariensis*.[80a]

HEDGE MUSTARD

Wireweed, Singer's Plant, Wild Mustard

Sisymbrium officinale

DISTRIBUTION Native to Europe and now worldwide. Naturalized in southern and eastern Australia.

HABITAT Found in cultivation, disturbed habitats and wasteland.

DESCRIPTION

Bristly annual or biennial herb growing to 60 cm (2 ft) with long, wiry stems branching almost at right angles.

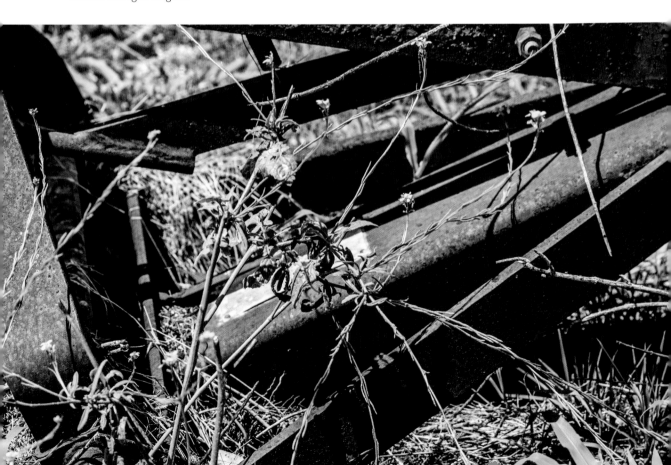

LEAVES Rosette of deeply divided leaves with toothed margins similar to Wild Turnip leaves. Leaves are coarse to the touch.

FLOWERS Tiny, pale yellow clusters growing terminally. Self-pollinates mainly in summer.

FRUIT/SEED Cone shaped fruit pods that lie flat against the branch with tapering tip.

USES

EDIBLE/OTHER Leaves and seeds used in salads, sauces and stews. In nineteenth century England, it was cultivated for this purpose. Leaves coarse so better cooked in stir-fries and soups. I often eat the flowers when foraging, they have a sweet and slightly peppery taste.

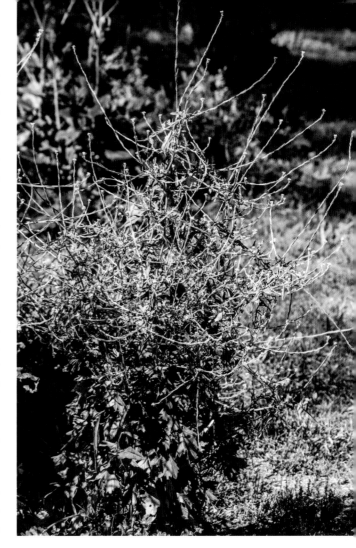

MEDICINAL When you see the word '*officinale*' in a botanical name it means it was in the seventeenth and eighteenth century an official medicine. Its value is due to its sulfurous volatile oils and it is specifically used for respiratory problems. Used to cure coughs, wheezing and loss of voice. In France was called 'Singer's plant' as the syrup was an infallible remedy for loss of voice in time of Louis XIV. Other uses as a diuretic, laxative, stimulant, stomachic and anticancer.

FARM/ENVIR. A weed of agricultural significance often found in cultivated fields. Suspected of tainting milk. Stock usually avoid eating this bristly plant. Attracts caterpillars and bees. This plant grows with other weeds and grasses on our property and I leave it growing, as like other Brassicas it is a good soil conditioner. Indicates soil very low in calcium, very high in potassium, magnesium, manganese, iron and other minerals. Low humus, bacteria, salty with good drainage.[8]

FURTHER READING Pharmacological and phytochemical study on a *Sisymbrium officinale* Scop. extract.[81] This study showed there was scientific basis for this plant's traditional uses.

HENBIT

Deadnettle

Lamium amplexicaule

DISTRIBUTION Native of Europe and Asia and now widespread. Naturalized throughout Australia especially the south-eastern region.

HABITAT Widespread weed of crops, gardens and disturbed areas.

DESCRIPTION

Annual, dainty herb grows up to 40 cm (16 in).

LEAVES Slightly hairy leaves with lobed margins growing opposite on darker square stems. Upper leaves are stem-clasping and lower leaves on long stalks.

FLOWERS Mauve-pink with a darker pink at the end of the flower tube that has two lip-like structures. Flowers grow in whorls widely spaced along the stem. Flowers in winter and early spring. Self-pollinates.

FRUIT/SEED 2,000 tiny seeds/plant.

USES

EDIBLE/OTHER Young leaves are cooked and used in various dishes or may be put into a green smoothie. It is a minor pot herb in Japan, Sweden and North America. Pick leaves before flowering.

MEDICINAL Has an astringent nature, good for any bleeding problems such as excessive menstruation, hemorrhaging and dysentery. As a 'blood purifier' good for rashes, eczema and an effective treatment for wounds, burns and bruises.

FARM/ENVIR. Competes with seedling vegetables and low growing crops. Will become an undesirable invasive plant if not properly managed. Sheep grazing on infested cereal stubble have developed 'staggers'. However once on good fodder they recover. Such a pretty little thing, I'm always delighted to find Henbit appearing in my vegetable patch as

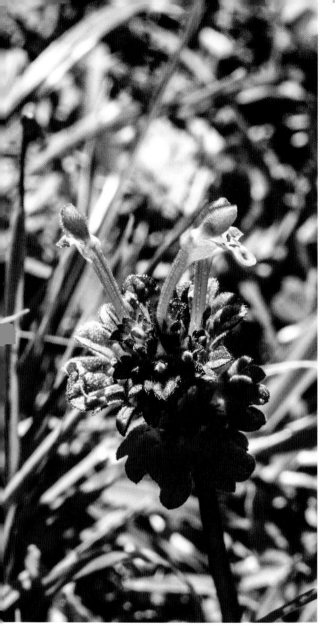
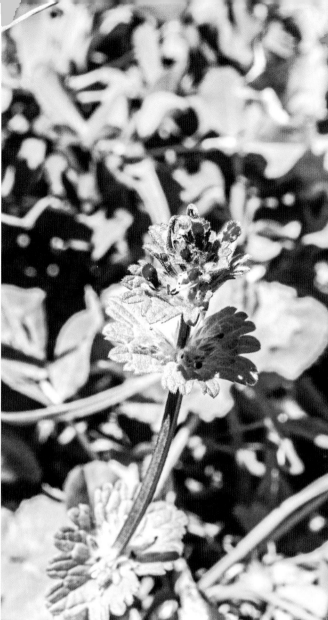

the ground warms up. Minor weed in the garden. Indicates soil low in calcium with poor humus, bacteria and sandy.[8]

MAY BE CONFUSED WITH Red Deadnettle (*L. purpureum*) which has furry leaves and upper leaves are on stalks. Has similar qualities.

FURTHER READING An inventory of the ethnobotanicals used as anthelmintics in the southern Punjab (Pakistan).[82] Analysis of the essential oil of *Lamium amplexicaule* L. from Northeastern Iran.[83]

WARNING Toxicity mainly in sheep fed on infested pastures.

HONEY LOCUST

Three-(t)horned Acacia, Bean Tree, Thorny Honey Locust

Gleditsia triacanthos

DISTRIBUTION Native to eastern North America and now a widespread species in subtropical and temperate regions throughout the world. Naturalized in southern and eastern Australia.

HABITAT Grows as a hardy forest tree in its native country but due to its invasive nature now creates dense thickets in pastures, disturbed sites, open woodlands and watercourses.

DESCRIPTION

Tall 15–30 m (50–100 ft), and wide thorny tree with branches and trunk covered in simple or branched spines up to 18 cm (7 in) long. Deciduous. Grows many suckers.

LEAVES Alternate leaves with numerous leaflets and finely toothed margins.

FLOWERS Inconspicuous, greenish or creamy-yellow borne on elongated drooping clusters. Flowers have a strong scent.

FRUIT/SEED Large, brown, flattened pods containing 15 to 25 large brown oval seeds surrounded by sweetish pulp, produced in autumn.

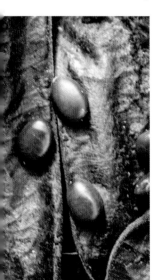

USES

EDIBLE/OTHER The young immature seeds may be eaten raw or cooked. They taste like young peas. Mature seeds can be roasted and ground as a coffee substitute. Mature and young pods are also cooked or made into a sweet-tasting drink. The pods have a sweet, fibrous, edible substance, which is pleasant to eat. Seeds are high in protein and carbohydrates. Other uses are for gum, tannin, thorns once used as nails, ornamental tree and generally useful wood.

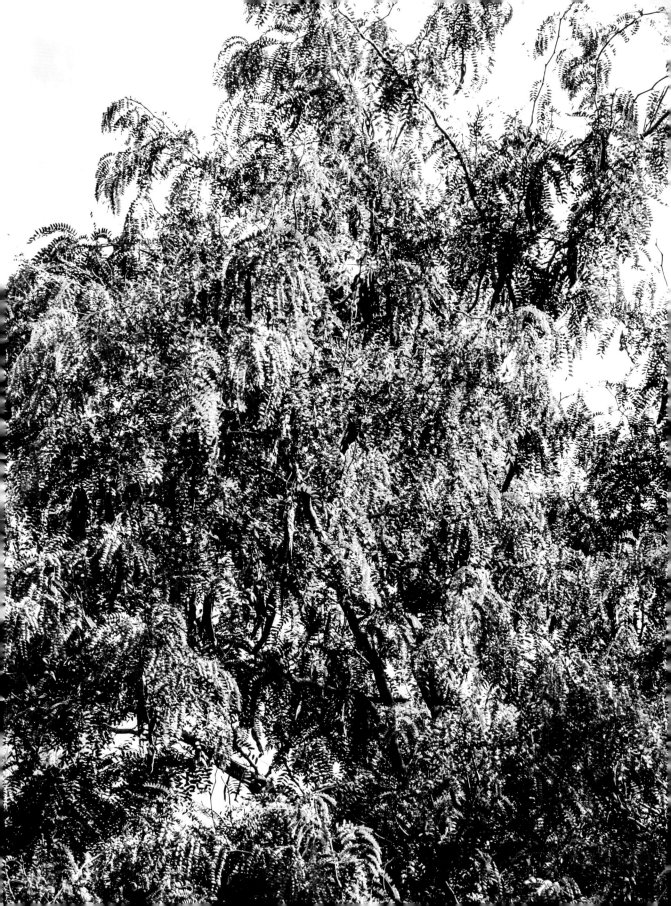

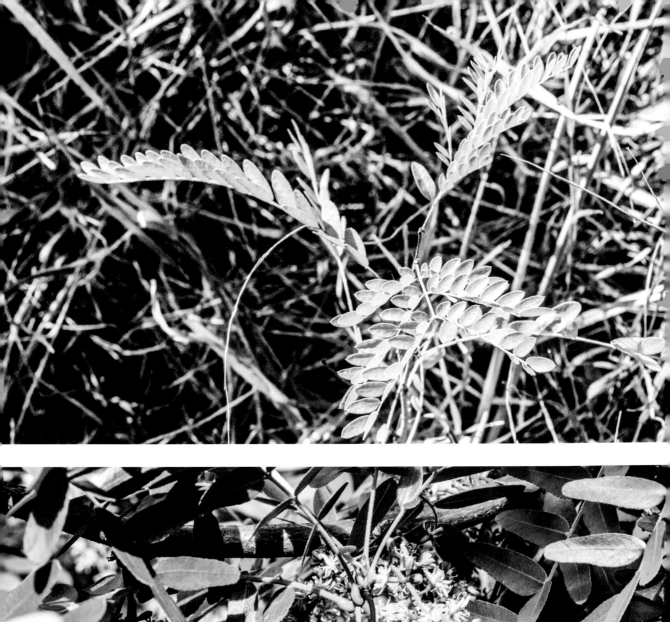
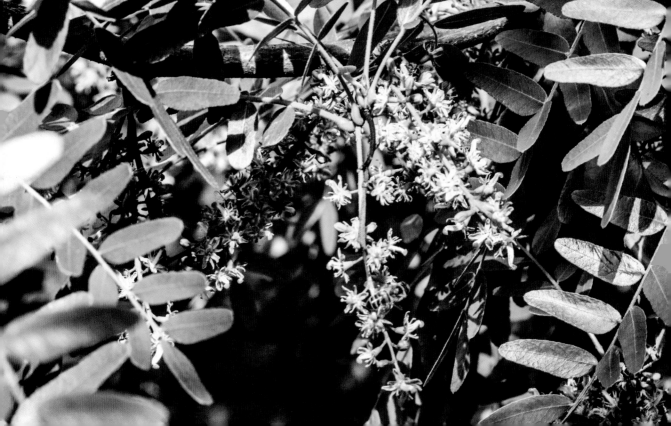

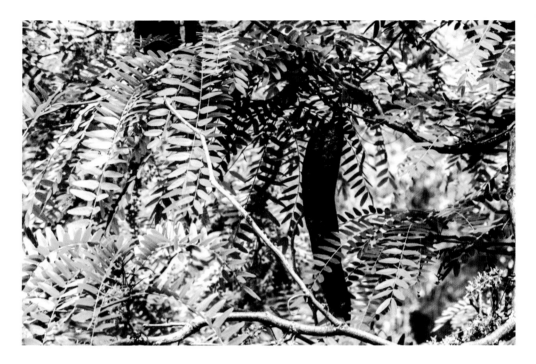

MEDICINAL Useful for pain, stomach problems, worming, tonic and an antiseptic. Use the pods for indigestion, measles, whooping cough, colds and other children's ailments. Bark for fever, measles, smallpox and upset stomach. Also a ceremonial plant.[84]

FARM/ENVIR. I have a majestic thorny tree in my orchard that I planted 30 years ago. I obtained a seedling from my parents' property where they had grown this tree on the recommendation of the Agricultural Department. It is a good fodder tree (especially the pods), hardy and very good for shade. In recent wetter seasons, I have noticed seedlings popping up near the tree and I dig them out with a hoe as it is classified as a noxious weed in New South Wales. It is an invasive exotic tree as it out-competes native vegetation. Its ability to sucker can create dense thick impenetrable thickets which smother productive grass species. Refuge for rabbits and foxes. Can be difficult and expensive to eradicate as thorns can inflict serious damage to people as well as their vehicles and equipment.[85] Pollutant tolerant tree, and used for reclamation of land. Also a good nitrogen fixer, and often grown as a nursery tree for orchards. Pods are high in nutrition for all livestock and wildlife.

FURTHER READING Evaluation of honey locust (*Gleditsia triacanthos* L.) gum as sustaining material in tablet dosage forms.[86] Analgesic activity of *Gleditsia triacanthos methanolic* fruit extract and its saponin-containing fraction.[87]

WARNING Contains some potentially toxic compounds. Beware of the thorns as they can inflict serious damage to stock and man.

HONEYSUCKLE, JAPANESE

Lonicera japonica

DISTRIBUTION Native of China, Japan and Korea now widely spread. Naturalized in southern and eastern Australia.

HABITAT This exotic species is found in neglected gardens, wasteland, gullies and river banks.

DESCRIPTION

Woody, twining climber with slender young branches.

LEAVES Oval to broad, lance-like.

FLOWERS Recognized by their distinctive trumpet like flowers of white and yellow with two lips. Flowers grow in the terminal leaf axis in pairs. Sweet scent. Flowers in summer

FRUIT/SEED Shiny, black, fleshy berry.

USES

EDIBLE/OTHER Suck nectar from flowers. Use the flowers in your vegetable or fruit salads and make a tea from the flowers and buds. Leaves can be cooked but contain high amount of saponins which are difficult to digest. Wild honeysuckle flowers are edible but avoid the ornamental varieties. Plant is a natural insecticide. Stems used to weave baskets.

MEDICINAL Popular in Chinese medicine for its antibacterial and anti-inflammatory properties. Used for fevers, headache, cough, sore throat and pain relief. Also used to lower blood pressure and blood cholesterol. Used externally to wash sores, inflammation and rashes.[89]

FARM/ENVIR. Aggressive vine, which develops a smothering mass of belowground runners and aboveground, intertwined stems that will cover extensive areas along the ground and into the canopy. It will smother native vegetation and cause havoc in orchards. A

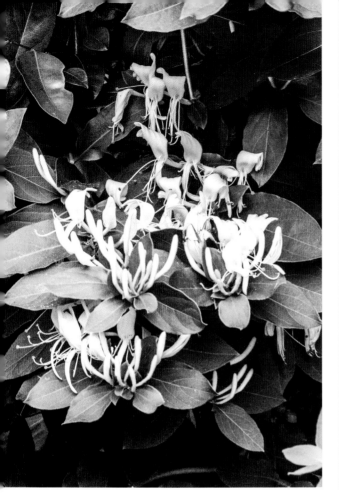
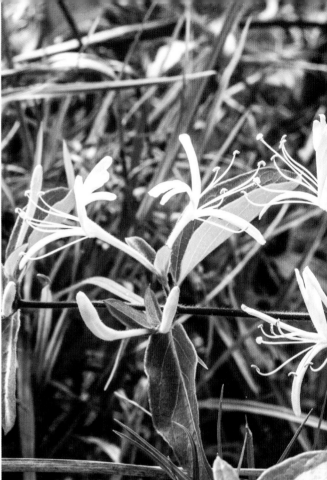

major pest in Australia and other countries. The first vine I found was growing in an old graveyard in Sydney and I've since found many more on creek banks. Avoid growing this aggressive vine and collect when needed from the wild. Better choice is the non-invasive Dutch honeysuckle. Indicates soil very low in calcium, phosphate and high in potassium, magnesium and copper. Low humus.[8]

MAY BE CONFUSED WITH There are over 100 species of honeysuckles and 12 would have medicinal value, most native to Eurasia. Dutch Honeysuckle (*L. periclymenum*) has edible flowers and has medicinal uses.

FURTHER READING Anti-inflammatory effect of the aqueous extract from *Lonicera japonica* flower is related to inhibition of NF-kappaB activation through reducing I-kappaBalpha degradation in rat liver.[88] The ethanol extract of *Lonicera japonica* (Japanese honeysuckle) attenuates diabetic nephropathy by inhibiting p-38 MAPK activity in streptozotocin-induced diabetic rats.[89] Antiangiogenic, antinociceptive and anti-inflammatory activities of *Lonicera japonica* extract.[90]

WARNING Berries toxic.

HOREHOUND

White Horehound, Common Horehound

Marrubium vulgare

DISTRIBUTION Native to Europe and the Mediterranean region and now widespread in temperate regions throughout the world. Naturalized throughout Australia especially the south-eastern region and declared noxious in some states.

HABITAT Adapted to poor, dry soils and has spread into pastures and wastelands.

DESCRIPTION

Erect, spreading, perennial herb growing to 75 cm (2 ft 6 in) in height having a woody base and dense white hairs that cover the square stems.

LEAVES Grey-green leaves have a crinkled surface with white hairs like down underneath the leaf.

FLOWERS Small white flowers grow in clusters around the stem.

FRUIT/SEED Flowers develop into a burr with hooked spines containing small seeds. Seeds mainly in summer.

USES

EDIBLE/OTHER Leaves are used as a seasoning — bitter and pungent. One of the six bitter herbs used in the Jewish Passover feast. An old and respected herb, ancient Romans loved it as a medicinal and magical herb. Horehound beer is a favorite and the tea is good for winter ills. Also a good honey plant.

MEDICINAL Popular in Europe as a folk remedy for curing coughs, colds and other respiratory problems. Especially for those dry, hacking, non-productive coughs, bronchitis, whooping cough and chesty colds. You can make lozenges, tea or syrups for immediate results. Being a strong bitter it also helps with diseases of the liver and gall. It helps with anemia, diabetes, high blood pressure, relieves pain, debility, delayed

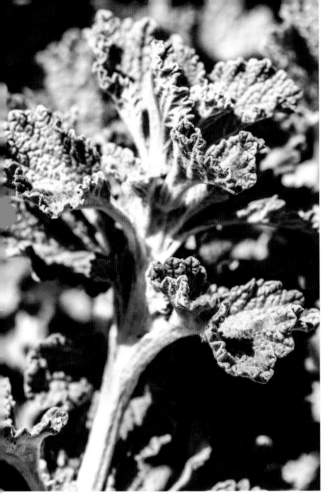
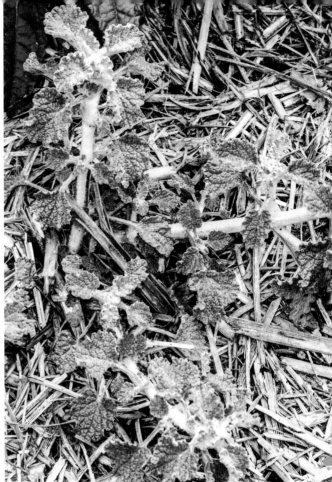

menstruation, nervous heart. Externally use as a compress for eczema and swollen glands especially in nervous and allergic types. Use a paste of the leaves for boils and rheumatism and powdered leaf as a mild disinfectant. A remedy I gave my children was to chop up a few leaves and have with honey at the first sign of sickness. The bitterness would scare any cold away.

FARM/ENVIR. A very unpopular herb with sheep and goat farmers because the burrs contaminate the wool and infest the whole property. Stock find Horehound unpalatable and it will taint the meat if the animals eat it. The juice used as a spray for canker worm in trees and as a fly spray. I have advised many students, if they put a few sprigs in their fruit trees, which have curly leaf, all the infected leaves will drop off. Then plant the herb underneath the tree. This works well.

FURTHER READING Comparative study of the antihypertensive activity of *Marrubium vulgare* and of the dihydropyridine calcium antagonist amlodipine in spontaneously hypertensive rat.[91] Analgesic potential of marrubiin derivatives, a bioactive diterpene present in *Marrubium vulgare* (Lamiaceae).[92]

INKWEED

Dye Berry

Phytolacca octandra

DISTRIBUTION Native to Mexico, Central and tropical America. It has spread to other tropical and subtropical countries. Grows throughout Australia especially north coast of New South Wales and Queensland.

HABITAT Growing in gardens, wastelands, newly cleared land, edge of native bushlands, parks and vacant lots. Prefers a good soil.

DESCRIPTION

Short-lived perennial small shrub, 1–3 meters (3–10 ft) high and readily distinguished by its spreading, smooth branched, red stems.

LEAVES Smooth, lance-like leaves grow on the thick stems changing from bright green in spring to reddish-purple in autumn.

FLOWERS Small, greenish-white flowers in dense spikes on short stalks.

FRUIT/SEED Numerous berries on the spike mature to a purple-black fleshy berry with reddish juice. Has eight slight lobes with eight small seeds.

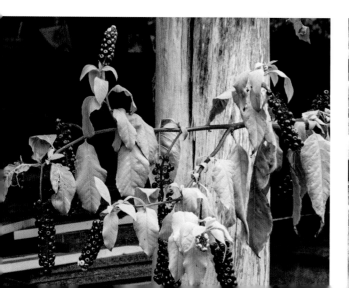
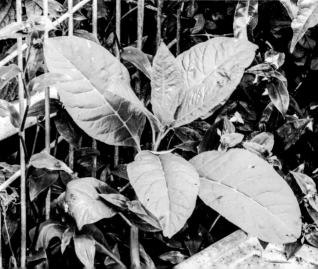

USES

EDIBLE/OTHER Inkweed is not edible. However closely related Poke Root (*P. Americana*) is eaten in dishes in America's south where generations of Appalachians celebrate Poke sallet season. Dye from the berries has been used to color alcoholic drinks and was used by children instead of ink.

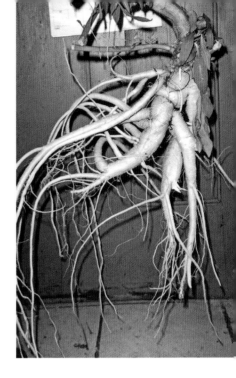

MEDICINAL I regularly dig up the roots of an Inkweed plant that must be two years or older and make an ointment or cream to help relieve sinusitis and related problems. The roots are used to make a compress for mastitis, tonsillitis, laryngitis, swollen glands and mumps. I also use Inkweed in my arthritis cream and use it externally on suspect sunspots. Overseas they eat the leaves and young stems to relieve diabetes and make a decoction of the roots for syphilis. It is advised not to take this herb internally until there is more research. This plant has been in Australia a long time as Aboriginal women told me that this herb was used for 'women's business' and an Aboriginal elder told me how he makes a brew from the leaves and stems to use it externally for any skin problem.

Its close relative Poke Root (*P. Americana*) is called herbal Drano and used for the lymphatic glands, chronic respiratory catarrh and chronic rheumatism. You can take this herb for internal use but only in minimal doses under direction.

FARM/ENVIR. A problem in some areas where it flourishes on newly cleared ground. Poisonous to stock, although they usually avoid it except for eating some berries. Birds love the berries. This plant is also a good soil builder with its deep taproot bringing up nutrients to the surface.

MAY BE CONFUSED WITH Poke Root (*P. Americana*) originating from the southern states of America. Has been recorded on the north coast of New South Wales and Queensland but is not common. Looks very similar but flowers grow on longer stalks with a less compact flower head, leaves more oval and fruit larger with 10 to 11 lobes and 10 to 11 seeds.

FURTHER READING Kaempferol-3-O-Ð-L-Arabinopyranosyl(1Ð6)-Ð-D-Galactopyranoside From *Phytolacca octandra* And Its Antimicrobial Activity.[93] A survey of antifungal compounds from higher plants, 1982–1993.[94]

WARNING Inkweed is both narcotic and poisonous, to be handled with great care and respect. Wear gloves when chopping up the root. When boiled the toxins are diminished. Suspected of poisoning stock.

ITALIAN THISTLE

Slender Thistle

Carduus pycnocephalus

DISTRIBUTION Native to Mediterranean region, western and southern Europe and now throughout the temperate zones of the world. Mostly found in the southern and eastern parts of Australia.

HABITAT Widespread weed of pastures, roadside, wasteland, stockyards, sheep camps, rabbit burrows and disturbed sites.

DESCRIPTION

Distinguished from other thistles by its relatively small flower heads. An erect annual herb 15–200 cm (6 in–6 ft 7 in) tall with a stout tap root. May produce many spiny green stems from the rosette.

LEAVES Rosette leaves often have conspicuous white patches along veins, upper leaves deeply lobed and covered in spines.

FLOWERS Solitary or two to five in terminal clusters, pink to rose-purple covered in spiny bracts. Flowers in spring/early summer.

FRUIT/SEED Small, long, tan-brown with relatively large pappus.

USES

EDIBLE Like most thistles, you can eat the stems by taking off the spiny rind but for its size, it would mainly be a survival food.

MEDICINAL Chinese medicine uses the plants of this family, treating colds, stomach-ache, rheumatism, inflammation, to relieve spasms, antiviral and antibacterial activity. Use as a dried herb, tincture or tea.

FARM/ENVIR. This noxious weed will grow into dense infestations smothering other smaller plants. It will limit access of livestock and cause physical damage as well as contaminating

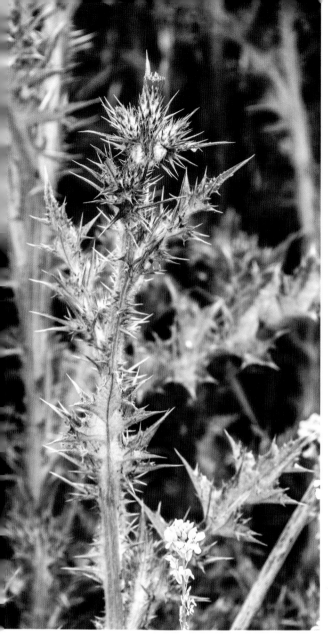
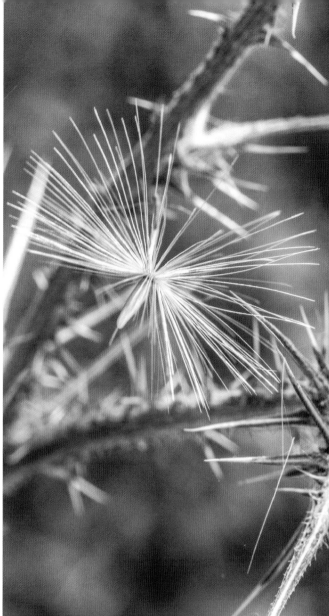

wool. It likes bare and disturbed sites and you can stop it propagating if there is reasonable ground cover. Graze with sheep, goats and horses to control it especially in autumn. I have noticed this plant dislikes competition – can be plentiful one year and minimal the next.

MAY BE CONFUSED WITH Slender Thistle (*Carduus tenuiflorus*) which is very similar except the Italian thistle has narrow, discontinuous wings along the stems. Often hybridized but seeds not very viable. Found in same regions in Australia.

FURTHER READING Anti-inflammation, antispasmodic use dried plant and for hypotensive activity use as a tea.[95]

JASMINE

Pink Jasmine, Chinese Jasmine and Winter Jasmine

Jasminum polyanthum

DISTRIBUTION Native to China and is widespread in many countries. Naturalized in south-eastern Australia.

HABITAT Garden escapee found in neglected gardens, wastelands, forests especially in wetter areas.

DESCRIPTION

Hardy fast growing perennial twining vine that can be trained to climb any surface.

LEAVES Leaflets with two to three pairs being dark green above and lighter green below.

FLOWERS Showy, delicate flowers with a distinctive scent. Flowers white on the outside and pink underneath. Flowers in spring.

FRUIT/SEED Small dark seeds.

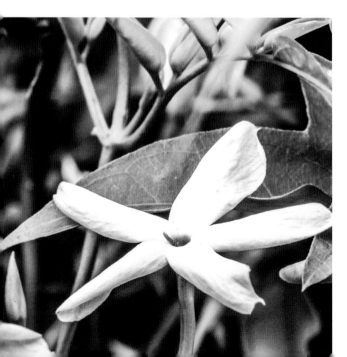

USES

EDIBLE/OTHER Flowers are edible, used as a garnish and in salads. Try sucking the nectar from the flowers, it is lovely and sweet. Add fresh or dried flowers to green tea to create your own mock Jasmine tea. There is even a recipe for a Jasmine tea infused vodka. Makes a lovely floral scent. Jasmine essential oil made from *J. officinale*.

MEDICINE In Chinese medicine several Jasmines are used for improving

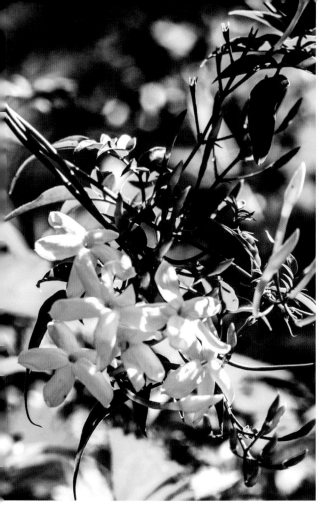
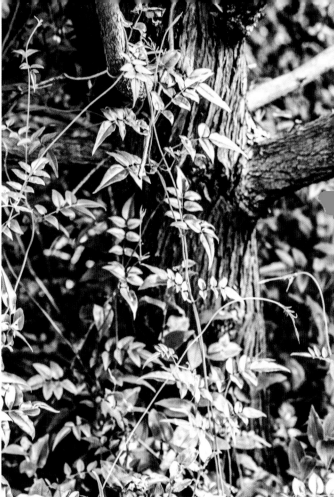

circulation, itchy skin, menstruation problems, pain relief and vaginal discharge. Also used for treatment of hepatitis, cirrhosis of the liver, discomfort of the chest, gastric pain, diarrhea, libido, tumors and abdomen pain. Make a decoction of the buds and flowers.

FARM/ENVIR. This plant is grown as an ornament and rarely a problem in cooler areas. However, in warmer, wetter climates this garden escapee has become a nuisance. Growing profusely, it will block out the light and restrict growth of natives. Serious weed in rainforests as it grows into the canopies. I have a massive plant that grows all over my fences and trees. I love its flowers and how it protects my natives but it has to be kept in check. I burn, hoe and cover with carpet to keep it managed. Edible and not poisonous to stock and pets.

MAY BE CONFUSED WITH There are 300 species in the genus *Jasminum* worldwide, 12 are Australian natives. All are trailing, climbing or erect shrubs. Exotic climbers which are grown for their showy, fragrant flowers.

FURTHER READING Jasmine (*Jasminum* spp.), westerlynaturalmarket.com.[96]

JERUSALEM ARTICHOKE

Sunroot

Helianthus tuberosus

DISTRIBUTION Native to North America and now growing worldwide. Naturalized mainly in eastern and southern Australia.

HABITAT Grows near habitation, along streams and into fields.

DESCRIPTION

Closely related to the cultivated sunflower. Renowned for its edible knobbly, fleshy roots that have grey, purple or pink skins. Stems are hairy and woody as they mature and develop many branches. Perennial but cultivated as an annual.

LEAVES Rough, oval to lance-like with coarsely toothed edges.

FLOWERS Bright yellow, flowering in summer. Center is a cluster of tiny yellow flowers surrounded by yellow 'petals'. Flowers in summer.

FRUIT/SEED Flowers will only develop seeds if pollinated by a different strain nearby. Seeds mottled black, flattened and wedge shaped. Mainly propagate by tubers.

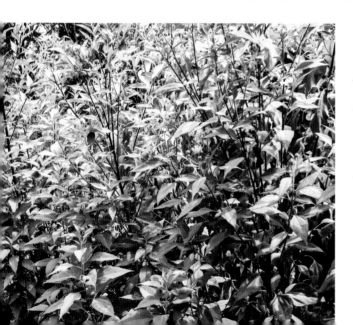

USES

EDIBLE/OTHER First grown by the American Indians for its edible, starch-rich tubers and then cultivated by early settlers. The tubers were taken overseas and grown widely as it is an easy crop to grow, hardy and quick growing. The sweet, ice-white, fleshy tubers are grated and eaten raw on salads or cooked like potatoes. As they contain inulin, an insoluble fiber this

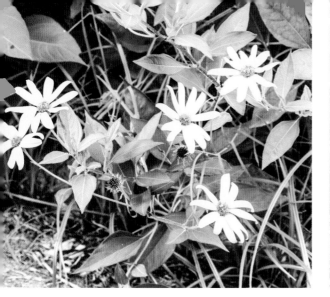 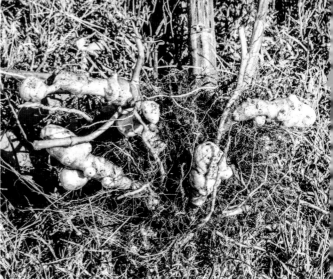

can be very hard for some people to digest and ferments in the gut causing severe wind. Inulin is converted to a natural sugar. Tubers roasted make a coffee substitute. I love this pretty plant and find the tubers sweet and crunchy but we all find them difficult to digest ('fartichokes').

MEDICINAL High in the oligofructose inulin which is a soluble non-starch polysaccharide so an ideal sweetener for diabetics. Contains 4% fiber. It also contains antioxidants and many minerals. New research is establishing the actions of this plant and proposing 10% Jerusalem Artichoke supplementation may be beneficial in the prevention of the onset of type 2 diabetes and non-alcoholic fatty liver disease.[97] The rhizomes are dried and ground to make a powder that is sold as a prebiotic and soluble fiber. I dry and grind the powder and make capsules with good results, helping nerve pain in the feet (peripheral neuropathy) especially clients who have diabetes type 2.

FARM/ENVIR. Escaped cultivation and grows in large stands. Use as a fodder crop in autumn. Especially good for pigs who love eating the roots. A source of biomass, it makes better alcohol than sugar beets and is very hardy and fast growing. My garden has large areas of Jerusalem Artichokes, which have grown from a few small tubers. If you wish to eradicate these plants by hand, you will need to remove every piece of tuber. Indicates soil high in magnesium, zinc, selenium and chloride. Poor humus, high moisture, poor drainage and a hardpan.[8]

MAY BE CONFUSED WITH Sunflower *(H. annuus)* a cultivated annual with larger flowers and tiny brown flowers in the center.

FURTHER READING Beneficial effects of soluble dietary Jerusalem Artichoke *(Helianthus tuberosus)* in the prevention of the onset of type 2 diabetes and non-alcoholic fatty liver disease in high-fructose diet-fed rats.[97] *Helianthus tuberosus* extract has antidiabetes effects in HIT-T15 Cells.[98]

KNOTWEED

Wireweed, Hogweed

Polygonum aviculare

DISTRIBUTION Cosmopolitan, naturalized throughout Australia.

HABITAT Weed of cultivation, found in wheat, Lucerne, pasture being established, wasteland and roadside.

DESCRIPTION

Much branched annual or short-lived perennial growing along the ground and easily identified in its mature state by long, wiry, stiff, smooth stems with swollen joints. Strong taproot.

LEAVES The joints are prominent, transparent, leafy out growths where the alternate, stalkless, lance-shaped or oval, blue-green leaves join the stem.

FLOWERS Minute, white to pale-pink flowers are in clusters of two or three in forks of the stem. Self-pollinating in summer.

FRUIT/SEED Copious tiny seeds that birds love.

USES

EDIBLE/OTHER The whole plant is edible and can be eaten raw or cooked or used in a tea. Eat in its younger stage as wiry when old. Edible seeds, related to buckwheat with similar uses. However, these seeds are so minute I would only use it as a survival food. Also used as a dye.

MEDICINAL A good astringent herb, good for diarrhea, bleeding piles, wounds and general bleeding. Good for kidney problems including kidney stones and fluid retention. Used to get rid of worms. An ointment made for sores and the juice squirted up the nose to stop it bleeding. In Ayurvedic and Unani medicine, this plant used as a laxative, stomachic, tonic, for fever and an antiseptic. Especially good for bacterial dysentery. Also an antioxidant.

FARM/ENVIR. Known as an environmental weed being a serious weed of crops and pastures as well as invading native vegetation. I remember this herb on the dairy farm where I grew up. It would grow in the Lucerne paddocks and when I was slashing with the tractor, its great long stems would tangle themselves around the blades. Not a favorite with farmers but is edible for stock. Once given to pigs when they were sick and they would recover quite quickly. Eradicate this weed by constant aeration and harrowing. Indicates soil very low in calcium, phosphate and very high in potassium, magnesium and selenium. Low humus, salty with poor drainage with hard crust and presence of aluminum.[8]

MAY BE CONFUSED WITH Buckwheat (*P. fagopyrum*), the only plant in this family that is cultivated for its edible seeds.

FURTHER READING The antiobesity effect of *Polygonum aviculare* L. ethanol extract in high-fat diet-induced obese mice.[99] Antioxidant activity of extract from *Polygonum aviculare* L.[100]

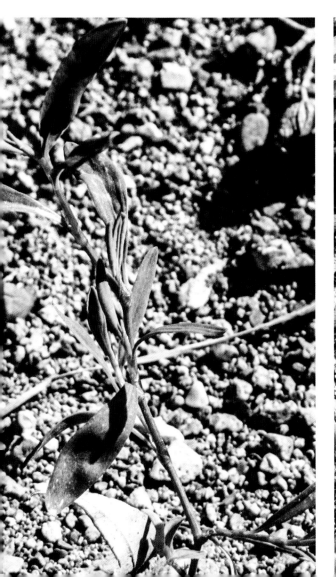

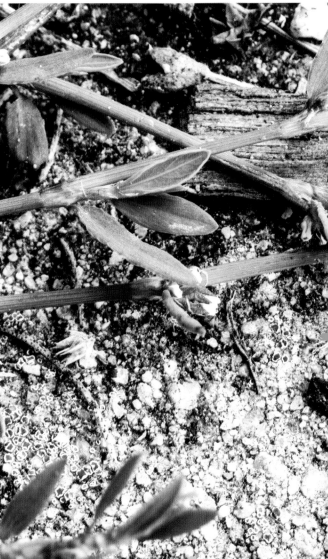

LANTANA

Prickly Lantana

Lantana camara

DISTRIBUTION Native to Central and South America and now widespread in many tropical and subtropical regions in the world. Naturalized in Australia especially the New South Wales and Queensland coastal regions.

HABITAT Inhabits cleared areas, rainforest margins, roadsides, parklands, along fence lines and wastelands.

DESCRIPTION

Much branched, erect, rambling shrub 2–4 m (6 ft 6 in) in height. Can grow like a vine up to 15 m (50 ft) into tree canopy. Branches are prickly and square in cross section.

LEAVES Opposite, oval with toothed margins with a rough texture.

FLOWERS Dense, flat-top clusters made up of numerous individual tubular flowers. They open from the outside inward and usually change color with age. Borne on stalks originally from leaf forks. Common colors are pink and red but there are numerous other colors in three circles of florets. One hundred different combinations in the wild varieties.

FRUIT/SEED Fleshy, purplish-black berry when ripe, has a single seed. Flowers and seeds throughout the year.

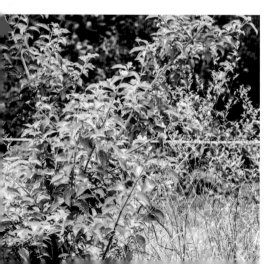

USES

EDIBLE/OTHER I have eaten the ripe fruits and found the soft black pulp surrounding the stone pleasant to eat. There is controversy about the fruits being edible, as children have died eating unripe fruits. Known as a survival food so eat minimal amounts. The stems are used in Africa to create products like cages for chooks. The coarse leaves are used as

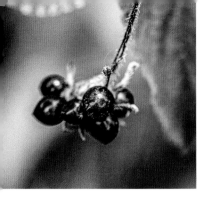
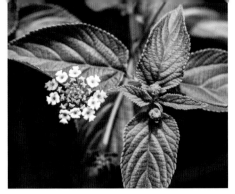
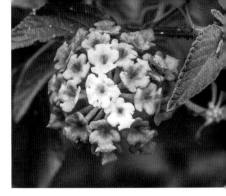

sandpaper for polishing fine-grained woods. In China, the stems were once fashioned into toothbrushes. Also makes a lovely floral arrangement and the dried leaves have a strong scent that can be used in potpourri.

MEDICINAL The boiled dried root is used internally for respiratory problems such as whooping cough and catarrhal infections; detoxifies, reduces fevers, used for mumps and skin problems. Burnt ash used to treat colds, coughs, toothache, sore throat and conjunctivitis. I have made an ointment from the tops of the plant and used it for skin problems such as chickenpox, psoriasis, rashes, bites, tinea and boils. Also used as a pesticide. New research is looking into using the essential oil and the flower extract in coconut oil to combat mosquitoes.[101, 102]

FARM/ENVIR. Nominated among 100 of the world's worst invaders by the International Union for Conservation of Nature Invasive Species Specialist Group. It is a most problematic, invasive and noxious plant throughout the world, especially Africa. Forms impenetrable thickets in forestry plantations, orchards, pasture land and invades natural areas. Spreads where humans have cleared land and fires have stimulated thicker growth. Fallen leaves produce a substance that prevents other plants from germinating and growing beneath, creating a monoculture. Birds and possums love the fruit but it may be toxic to stock. Hard to eradicate by natural means, best is early detection and response. Biocontrol is the only long-term and sustainable method of control. Make a spray from the plant and use on fruit to control bacterial, viral and fungal diseases. Crushed leaves used on animals for cuts and wounds. Indicates soil very low in calcium, phosphate and very high in potassium, iron and high in magnesium and manganese. Poor humus and sandy soil.[8]

MAY BE CONFUSED WITH Creeping lantana (*L. montevidensis*) which is similar to *L. camara* except it is a prostate form with no prickles.

FURTHER READING Repellency of *Lantana camara (Verbenaceae)* flowers against Aedes mosquitoes.[101] Adulticidal activity of essential oil of *Lantana camara* leaves against mosquitoes.[102] Antibacterial activity of *Lantana camara* Linn and *Lantana montevidensis* Briq extracts from Cariri-Ceará, Brazil.[103]

WARNING Has been known to poison children (unripe fruit) and when eaten in large amounts toxic to stock. Beware when collecting as may have been sprayed with herbicide.

LEMON BALM

Common Balm, Beebalm, Melissa

Melissa officinalis

DISTRIBUTION Native to southern and central Europe and the Mediterranean region and now growing widespread. Naturalized in south-eastern Australia especially Victoria and Tasmania.

HABITAT Grown for its scent and usage, now a garden escapee. Growing in gardens, near habitation, wasteland and beside creeks. Likes nutrient rich soils, adequate rainfall and a sunny position.

DESCRIPTION

Perennial, growing up to 60 cm (2 ft) on short rootstock. Has a slightly hairy, square stem, branching near the top.

LEAVES Greenish-yellow, opposite, oval with serrated edges. Distinct lemon scent.

FLOWERS Usually white but occasionally pinkish or yellow. Small flowers appear late summer to mid-autumn.

FRUIT/SEED Fruit is dry but does not split open when ripe.

USES

EDIBLE/OTHER Use the leaves as a flavoring agent. Lemon Balm cheesecake is popular with my students and my favorite tea contains this calming herb. Put the chopped leaves in your next salad, in your juice or my favorite is in a fruit platter. Lemon Balm is an ingredient in potpourri, herb pillows, bath bags, in licorice and wines. An essential oil from the leaves is good for many problems. A very good bee plant.

MEDICINAL Used for hundreds of years as a calming, relaxing herb, excellent for melancholy. Use to relieve spasms, lower blood pressure, helps colic, digestive problems, dizziness, fever, flu, headache, cold sores, hyperthyroidism, insect bites, insomnia, menstruation, morning sickness, nausea, nerves, restlessness, nightmares, palpitations, PMT, sedative, antiviral and for dressing wounds. I preserve a juice of the leaves and find it very effective for calming children.

FARM/ENVIR. Only grows in certain localities in Australia so only a minor weed. Commercial cultivation of this plant is viable as it has a growing market. Stock will eat this plant. In winter my plants die down with the frost but quickly grow when the weather warms.

FURTHER READING Antimicrobial and antioxidant activities of *Melissa officinalis* L. (Lamiaceae) essential oil.[104] *Melissa officinalis* extract in the treatment of patients with mild to moderate Alzheimer's disease.[105] Local therapy of herpes simplex with dried extract from *Melissa officinalis*.[106]

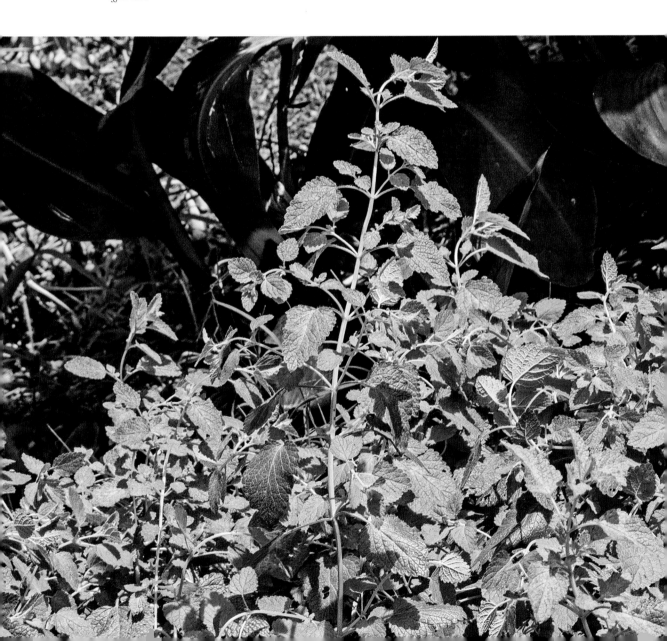

LUCERNE

Bastard Medic, Alfalfa

Medicago sativa

DISTRIBUTION Native to Asia and now widely distributed in temperate zones of the world as popular in agriculture. Naturalized throughout Australia.

HABITAT Growing as a weed on roadsides, riverbanks and wasteland.

DESCRIPTION

Long-lived, erect perennial, 1 m (3 ft 3 in) high with a deep taproot.

LEAVES Alternating up the stem composed of three lance-like to oval, blue-green leaflets.

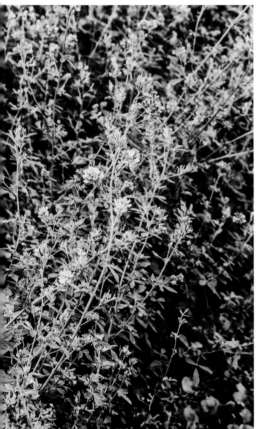

FLOWERS Borne in loose clusters with five petals, colored purple, violet, pink, white or yellow. Flowers late summer to mid-autumn.

FRUIT/SEED Pods sickle to a spiral shape. Each pod contains several kidney-shaped seeds.

USES

EDIBLE/OTHER Leaves and young shoots are cooked in dishes or dried for tea and can be ground into a powder as a health supplement. The seeds can be ground and eaten as a health food or sprouted (alfalfa sprouts). High in protein, calcium and other vitamins and minerals. Controversy about the toxins found in the leaves and seeds. They contain saponins, which are hard to digest, may cause gas due to incomplete digestion. There is also a toxic substance found in the seeds called canavanine sulfate (2%) which is the plant's protective defense

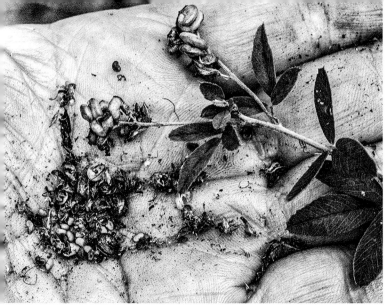 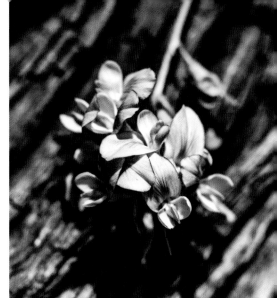

against insects, animals and microorganisms. However, research shows that having small amounts of alfalfa sprouts daily does not represent a health hazard as the body can move toxins away. Except for people with diseases like lupus who should avoid the sprouts and seeds.[107]

MEDICINAL Herbal medicine for 1,500 years. Good for making mother's milk and a general tonic. American Indians heated the leaves and used for earache; Chinese for digestive tract and kidneys; Indians for poor digestion, fevers, tonic, kidney stones, antibacterial, arthritis and water retention. Also used for anemia, diabetes, appetite, PMT, diuretic and to lower cholesterol. I use the dried leaves and flowers to make a pleasant alkaline tea.

FARM/ENVIR. This was the first forage crop to be domesticated and now there are many pest resistant cultivars. I have childhood memories of fragrant Lucerne, contented dairy cows, abundant milk and the smell of freshly cut Lucerne hay. I also remember that my father had to spray the Lucerne to stop bloat in the cattle. It makes excellent hay and now farmers also harvest the plant and seed for human consumption. The leaf meal is used to fortify baby food and other special dietary food. Also used in manufacturing concentrated feed for livestock and poultry. Most domesticated and wild animals and birds love grazing on this crop. It has become a weed in some regions and habitats and can become invasive displacing other vegetation if not properly managed.

FURTHER READING Evaluation of antioxidant and cerebroprotective effect of *Medicago sativa* L. against ischemia and reperfusion insult.[108]

WARNING Alfalfa sprouts have caused food poisoning from salmonella and E. coli and there is a recommendation from the US Food and Drug Administration to cook sprouts before eating. Also avoid if you have any lupus-like symptoms.

MALLOW

Marshmallow, Small Flowered Mallow

Malva parviflora

DISTRIBUTION Native to the Mediterranean region and Europe and now growing worldwide. Naturalized throughout Australia.

HABITAT Grows on all soil types and found in old sheepyards, near farm buildings, roadsides, cultivation, wasteland and degraded pastures.

DESCRIPTION

Erect sprawling herb with small stiff hairs and a strong taproot. Grows up to 1 m (3 ft 3 in) in height and has a woody base. Grows in large numbers in the cooler months.

LEAVES Rounded with scalloped margins and radiating veins.

FLOWERS Small, pale pink to white with five petals that are barely bigger than the green, cup-shaped calyx that encloses the flower.

FRUIT/SEED Seedpods look like buttons or cheeses and they split into eight to twelve wedge-shaped segments when ripe.

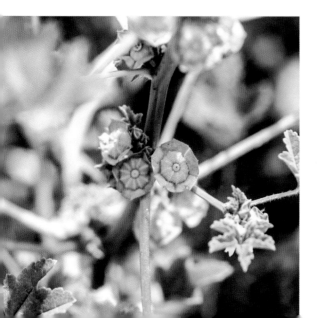

USES

EDIBLE/OTHER After autumn or winter rains my garden is a mass of majestic Mallow plants and I use them for many purposes. Most Mallows are edible and the young stems, leaves, flowers and seedpods can be eaten raw or cooked. They contain mucilage, which is a natural thickener so if cooked in soups, stews, sauces or other dishes will act like Okra (closely related) and thicken the dish. Also makes a soothing tea.

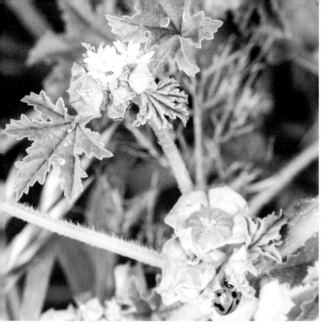
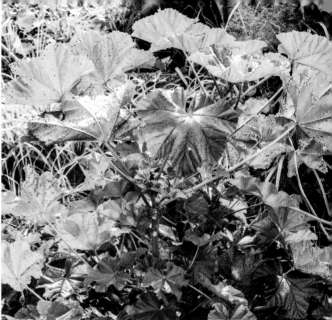

MEDICINAL Being rich in slimy mucilage it makes an excellent tea or tincture to sooth sore throats, coughs, ulcers in the bladder, stomach ulcers and stomachaches. This herb has little taste so add peppermint leaves or lemon and honey. Externally, use the leaves to make a compress, poultice or make into a cream or ointment to use on abscesses, boils, wounds, minor burns and insect bites. It is one of the ingredients in my Cure-all weed ointment and cream. The mucilage forms a protective film over inflamed mucous membranes internally and externally. Has anti-inflammatory and antioxidant properties. Widely used in Africa as a medicinal herb growing on heavily grazed grassland.

FARM/ENVIR. Mallows belong to a group of weeds that follow human steps and cultivation. Roots delve down penetrating deep clays and aerating the soil thus making an excellent plant for reclaiming compacted soils. I've seen them covering cowyards with soils so downtrodden that nothing else will grow. Years later those yards are covered in thick grass. Definitely one of nature's little helpers. However, not liked by farmers as this plant can cover large areas and if sheep are locked in these paddocks with little other feed they can develop staggers. Animals will eat this plant but prefer other pastures. Indicates soil very low in calcium, very high in magnesium, high in potassium, iron and selenium. Low humus with a hardpan.[8]

MAY BE CONFUSED WITH Dwarf Mallow (*M. neglecta*) which has flowers twice as long as the calyx and Tall Mallow (*M. sylvestris*) with its much larger, attractive, pink-mauve flowers. Both mallows are used the same as *M. parviflora*. The true Marshmallow (*Althea officinalis*) growing in Europe is more renowned for its medicinal actions.

FURTHER READING Variation in antibacterial and anti-inflammatory activity of different growth forms of *Malva parviflora* and evidence for synergism of the anti-inflammatory compounds.[109]

MUGWORT, CHINESE

Chinese mugwort

Artemisia verlotorum

DISTRIBUTION Native to China and surrounding countries and spread to Eurasia, South America and Oceania. Naturalized in Australia in eastern coastal and subcoastal areas and Victoria.

HABITAT Prefers moist sites such as riverbanks, waterways, vegetation, swampy and disturbed areas.

DESCRIPTION

An erect perennial aromatic herb growing up to 1 m (3 ft 3 in) in height. Has long creeping rhizomes, which can dominate upper soil layers.

LEAVES Green above and grey-white underneath. Upper leaves elongated with many deeply dissected. Leaves are variable.

FLOWERS Inconspicuous yellowish to reddish-brown in color with a pleasant aroma. Profuse and very leafy flowering late summer.

FRUIT/SEED Usually not produced. Mainly reproduces by rhizomes.

USES

EDIBLE/OTHER Chinese use this plant to flavor dishes. However, due to its toxicity mainly use Common Mugwort. Has insecticidal properties.

MEDICINAL Used as a medicinal herb for the respiratory, circulatory and digestive systems. Careful administration is important as large amounts are potentially toxic. Roots used to make moxibustion sticks used in traditional Chinese medicine. Common Mugwort mainly used. Essential oil shows antimicrobial activity mainly against yeast.[110]

FARM/ENVIR. I found a dense stand of this herb growing beside a nearby river. It is an environmental weed in many water systems. As it spreads by underground rhizomes and forms large, dense colonies it has the ability to influence the structure and behavior of rivers. Its stands are so thick that it smothers other ground cover plants and prevents regeneration of native trees and shrubs. Livestock usually avoid grazing on this plant as it is bitter. Indicates soil very low in calcium, high in magnesium with low humus.[8]

MAY BE CONFUSED WITH Common Mugwort (*A. vulgaris*) is closely related to Chinese Mugwort and has many medicinal actions. It differs by having very little aroma, does not grow in such strong stands, has viable seeds and its leaves are shorter. Also related to Wormwood (*A. absinthium*) a medicinal herb with its silvery leaves and yellow flower heads.

WARNING Major hayfever causing plant. Large amounts have a genotoxic potential.[111] May cause contact dermatitis in sensitive individuals. Toxic to stock in large amounts.

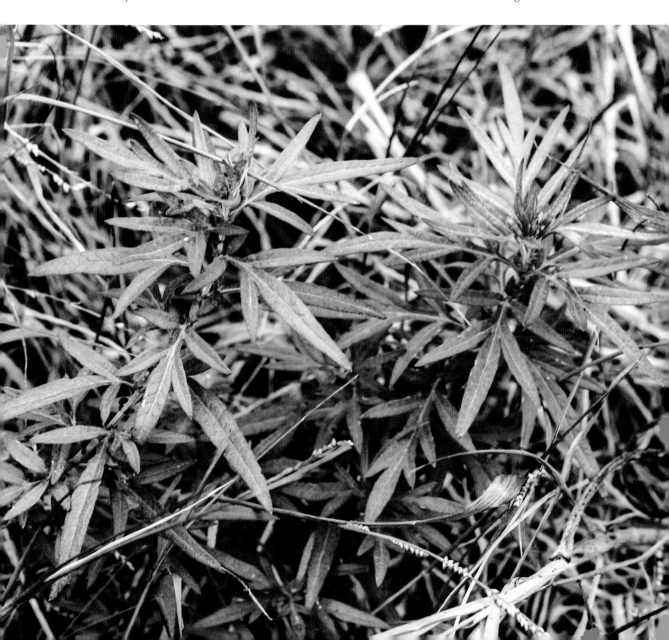

MULLEIN

Great Mullein, Aaron's Rod, Velvet Plant

Verbascum thapsus L.

DISTRIBUTION Native of Europe and Asia and now widespread in temperate regions of the world. Naturalized in south-eastern Australia.

HABITAT Commonly seen on roadsides, rocky slopes, uncultivated fields and degraded pastures. Grows in the cooler areas in our district.

DESCRIPTION

Erect perennial or biennial robust herb up to 2 m (6 ft 6 in) high. Whole plant covered in woolly white hairs giving the plant a velvety appearance.

LEAVES A rosette of bluish-green, velvet-looking leaves appear before a stem appears then leaves taper to the base to form wings on the stem. Leaves long and ovate.

FLOWERS Creamy, yellow flowers grow up the stem with white hairs on the stamen. Flowers in spring and early summer.

FRUIT/SEED Small prolific seeds that have a long life.

USES

EDIBLE/OTHER Flowers and leaves are edible but best used in tea. Roman ladies would use the flowers to dye their hair yellow. Plant creates various dyes. Leaves placed in shoes used to help circulation and keep feet warm. When dried makes excellent tinder, and used as lamp wicks.

MEDICINAL Traditionally used for respiratory problems especially where there is a dry hard cough and helps to bring up mucus. Research has shown good results for chronic earache using a combination of infused oils of Mullein, Garlic, Calendula and St John's Wort. It also has antiviral action against the influenza virus, has antibacterial, antitumor

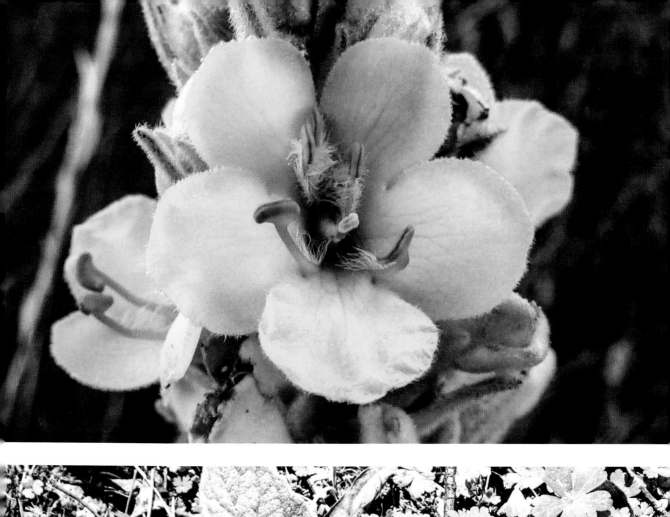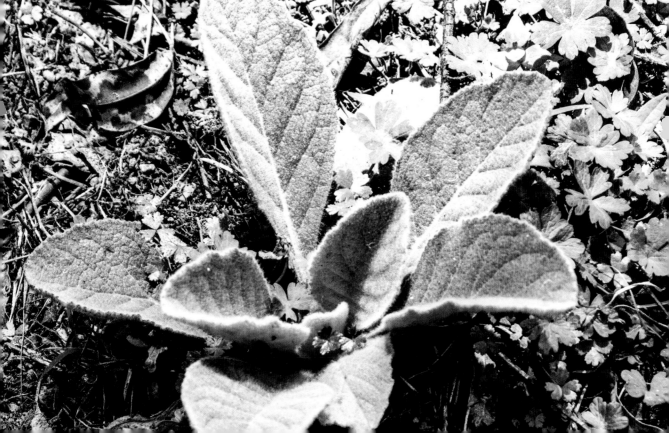

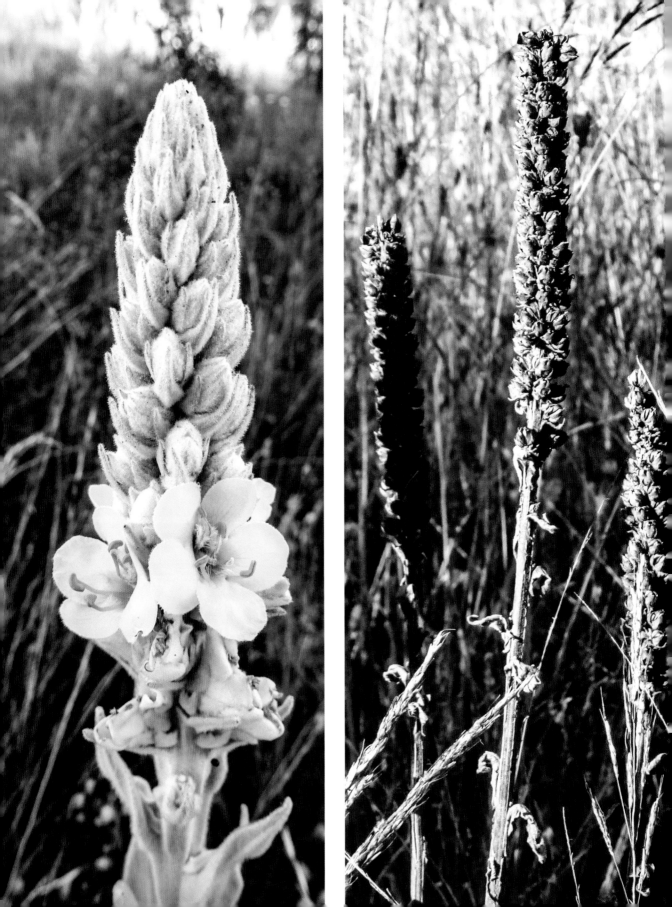

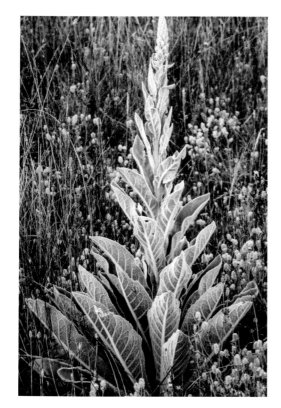
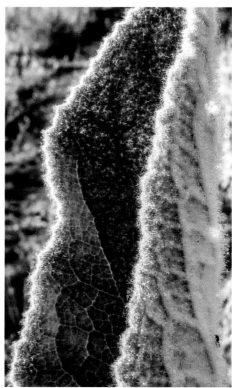

and antioxidant properties. Good activity against round and tapeworms. High mucilage content makes it excellent for various skin problems.[112]

FARM/ENVIR. Livestock are not fond of the irritating, hairy foliage. The leaves used for cattle – diarrhea and cattle cough. Insects love the flowers, which are high in pollen and nectar. When I walk the hills in the cooler areas, I see these plants dotted around the paddocks and clinging to the stony rocky hills. It can grow in thick stands in some areas and needs management. However, it is not very competitive and cannot survive tilling. Indicates soil very low in calcium, phosphate and very high in potassium, magnesium, sodium, zinc and selenium. Low humus and moisture with good drainage and sandy soil.[8]

MAY BE CONFUSED WITH Twiggy Mullein (*V. virgatum* Stokes) which is a widespread weed, growing locally, growing like Mullein except it has no woolly hairs. Its flowers are yellow with purple hairs on the stamens. Used in Spain for respiratory and cardiovascular problems.

FURTHER READING Common Mullein (*Verbascum thapsus* L.): recent advances in research [113] Anthelmintic and relaxant activities of *Verbascum thapsus* Mullein.[114]

NASTURTIUM

Indian Cress

Tropaeolum majus

DISTRIBUTION Native of South America now widespread worldwide. Naturalized in Australia in coastal districts and south-eastern regions.

HABITAT Unkempt gardens, wastelands, watercourses, urban bushland, roadsides, railways and disturbed sites especially around towns.

DESCRIPTION

Short-lived creeping or sprawling plant with somewhat fleshy stems. Dies down with frosts.

LEAVES Distinctive circular, spirally arranged leaves borne on long stalks attached to the center.

FLOWERS Bright, attractive, trumpet-shaped colored red, orange or yellow. Prominent nectar spurs at the base. Flowers in the warmer months.

FRUIT/SEED Three-celled, capsular, green, succulent fruit.

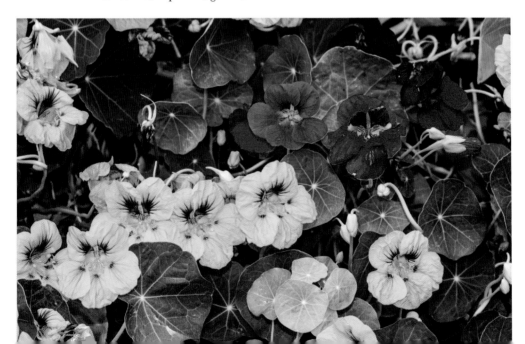

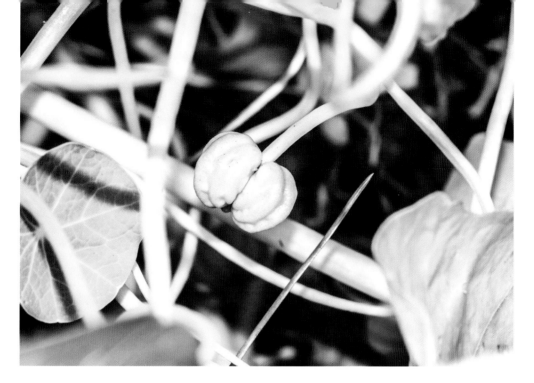

USES

EDIBLE/OTHER Flowers and young leaves are a spicy cress substitute, delicious in salads, sandwiches or cooked dishes. The flowers add color. Try stuffing the leaves and flowers with cottage cheese, then sprinkle with paprika, a great favorite of mine. Use the green seeds as a caper substitute. Only plant other than those in the Mustard family that contains mustard oil. However, the peppery taste is not noticeable unless chopped or chewed. Whole plant is very nutritious high in sulfur, iodine, potassium, phosphate and Vitamin C. Grow as a pretty, ornamental and useful plant.

MEDICINAL An exclusive remedy for two main systems, the respiratory and urinary. Contains Benzyl isothiocyanate, which inhibits or kills gram-positive and negative bacteria and fungi. Reduces mucus, helps to bring up phlegm and used externally for acne and skin problems.[115] In Germany one firm makes a heart remedy of Nasturtium. Seeds contain the strongest mustard oil: make into a fresh juice or into powder to treat staphylococcus, salmonella and streptococcus.

FARM/ENVIR. Once a popular, low-maintenance garden plant but no longer fashionable. Has escaped cultivation and now an environmental weed. Good companion plant for fruit trees. Put deterrents around your brassicas and the white butterfly will eat the Nasturtiums. Good ground cover and attracts many useful insects.

FURTHER READING Antihypertensive effects of isoquercitrin and extracts from *Tropaeolum majus* L.: evidence for the inhibition of angiotensin converting enzyme.[116] Evaluation of subchronic toxicity of the hydroethanolic extract of *Tropaeolum majus* in Wistar rats.[117]

NETTLES

Dwarf or English *(Urtica uren)*, Common or Tall Nettle *(Urtica dioica)*, Scrub or Native Nettle *(Urtica incisa)*

DISTRIBUTION English Nettle is cosmopolitan and grows worldwide. Naturalized in Australia in the southern and eastern regions. Tall Nettle is cosmopolitan and grows worldwide. Naturalized on the coast of New South Wales, also Victoria and Tasmania. Scrub Nettle is native to Australia and found mainly in south-eastern Australia.

HABITAT Nettles like moist fertile areas, paddocks, crops, creek banks, pastures, farms and along rainforest margins.

DESCRIPTION

Erect plants identified by the rigid stinging hairs that cover the leaves and stems. Root and rhizome long, creeping and yellowish. English Nettle is a small, annual plant with 5 cm (2 in) long ovate leaves and the male and female flowers are together in one flower head. Grows in the cooler months in shady, cool areas. Tall Nettle is perennial, taller 25–100 cm (10 in–3 ft 3 in) with opposite, ovate leaves and male and female flowers on separate plants. Scrub Nettle is a taller perennial with lance like leaves up to 10 cm (4 in) long and usually male and female flowers are on separate plants.

LEAVES Oval to lance-like leaves with serrated margins and covered in stinging hairs.

FLOWERS Sprays of small, greenish flowers. Flower in the warmer months.

FRUIT/SEED Small seeds high in oil.

USES

EDIBLE/OTHER Nettles are excellent for eating. The Nettle bed was common place in the English country garden. It was the first green vegetable in spring and sold in eighteenth century markets. High in chlorophyll and nutrients, excellent in any recipe that requires greens. Pick the young leaves and always wear gloves If you get stung do not rub or it will cause a histamine reaction that can last for days. Use dock, plantain, bracken or juice from

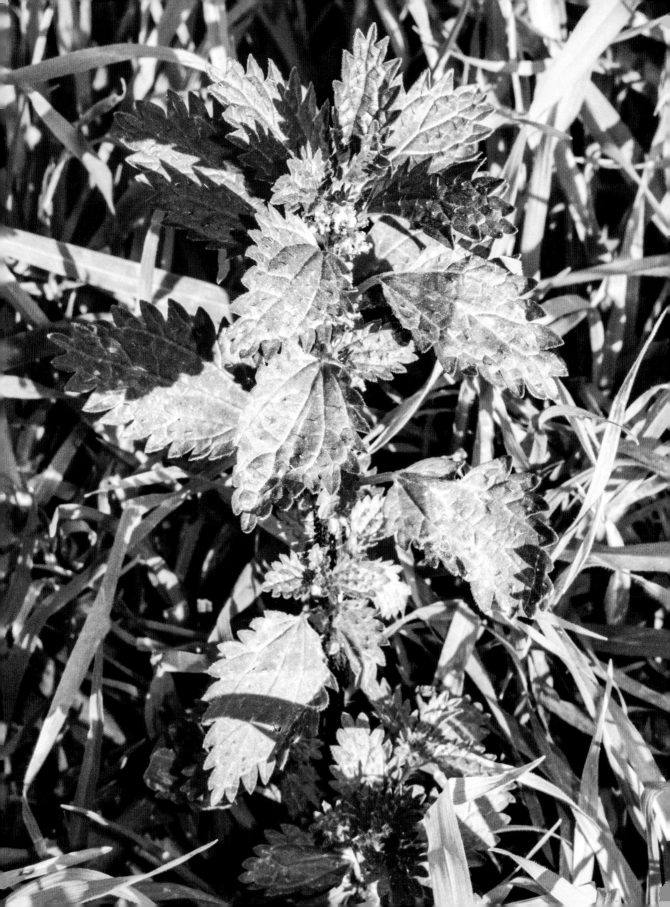

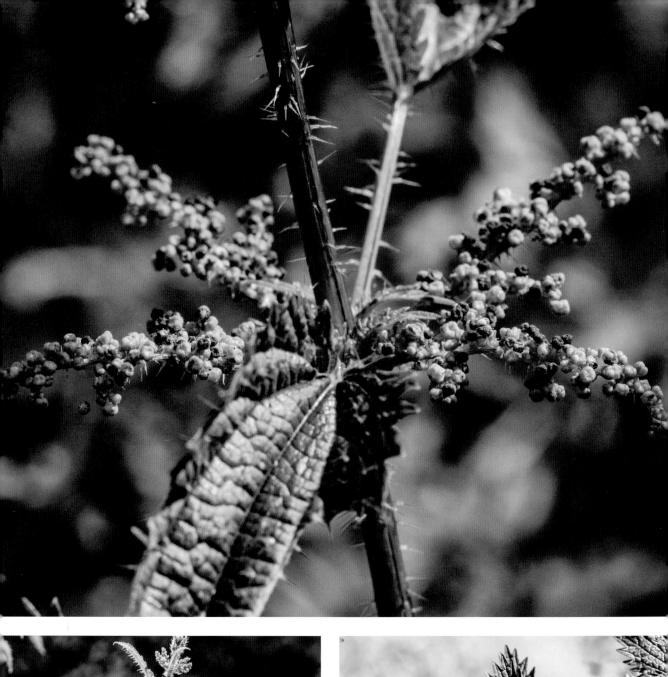
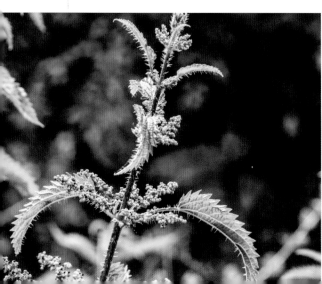
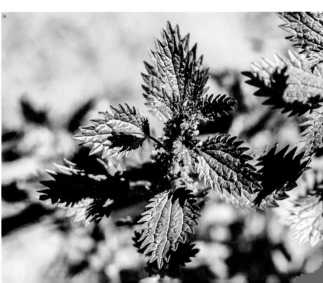

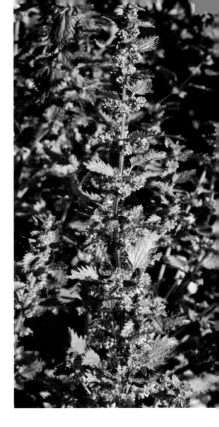

the Nettle itself to relieve the sting. I dry and crush the Nettles to make Nettle quiche and use them in soups. The crushed seeds have enough oil to run lamps. The fiber is used to weave cloth and leaves and roots to make dye. My favorite use, as a hair conditioner. Tonic for the scalp and strengthens the hair follicles. Nettle beer still an old favorite.

MEDICINAL Being a storehouse in minerals, it strengthens the whole body. Research has shown that it is specific for benign enlarged prostate. Useful for inflammation, allergic rhinitis, osteoarthritis, blood cleanser, stops bleeding, treats diarrhea, dysentery, chronic diseases of the colon and blood sugar disorders. Used externally for gout, sciatica, joint pain, skin problems such as eczema, nettle rash and skin eruptions. Seeds for goiter and good to make mother's milk. An antioxidant, good herb for the liver and the heart.[118] The syrup is for bronchial and asthmatic problems. Topically, use in an ointment or cream for skin problems and insect bites. It is one of the ingredients in my Cure-all weed ointment and cream. I also use it as an extract, tincture, ground as a powder and in tea and capsules. As a tea it has very absorbable silica. Europeans and Australian Aborigines both used Nettles to practice urtication (flogging with Nettles) as a treatment for rheumatism, muscular stiffness, sciatica, paralysis and gout. Drink Nettle tea regularly to keep free from disease. Add other herbs for flavor such as peppermint or lemon.

FARM/ENVIR. Stock will eat Nettles mainly when very young or when they go to seed. In Russia and Sweden the plant is cultivated as a fodder plant being mown several times a year to feed cattle. Horses' coats shine when nettle seeds are added to their oats. Dried and powdered Nettle in poultry food increases egg production and dried Nettle hay fed to dairy cows increases milk production. Turkeys and pigs also fatten on this weed. In the garden and pastures it has good dynamic characteristics: plants grow more resistant; neighboring crops change their chemical process e.g. peppermint increases its oil content and Nettle roots stimulate humus formation. Excellent in the compost or use as a complete fertilizer. You can also spray the tea on plants to keep them healthy. English Nettles indicate soil low in calcium, very low in phosphate and very high in potassium, magnesium, iron and copper. Low humus, bacteria and hard crust.[8]

FURTHER READING *Urtica dioica* for treatment of benign prostatic hyperplasia: a prospective, randomized, double-blind, placebo-controlled, crossover study.[119] Effects of *Urtica dioica* extract on lipid profile in hypercholesterolemic rats.[120]

WARNING Stinging hairs can cause irritation and redness.

NOOGOORA BURR

Cockle Burr

Xanthium occidentale

DISTRIBUTION Native to Americas now growing worldwide. Naturalized throughout Australia. *X. occidentale* is a subspecies of *X. strumarium*.

HABITAT Weed of crops, cultivation, pastures, waterways, roadsides, disturbed areas. Grows in various environments and after flooding it will occupy large areas of pasture and range lands.

DESCRIPTION

Xanthium species are robust annual herbs and they have distinctive spiny fruits. X. occidentale is an upright, spreading, short-lived plant up to 1 m (3 ft 3 in) in height. Much-branched stems covered in short, stiff hairs that give them a rough texture.

LEAVES Maple-leaf shaped – large, broad, irregularly-toothed leaves, which are rough.

FLOWERS Indistinct separate male and female flower heads produced on different regions of the branches. Flowers in the summer.

FRUIT/SEED Oval shaped burr containing two seeds. Fruit covered in numerous hooked spines and two larger spines at the top.

USES

EDIBLE/OTHER Contains toxins but in some cultures the young leaves and tender tops are used as a vegetable. Makes a yellow dye. Seeds yield a lamp oil.

MEDICINAL Ayurvedic and Sidha medicine use the very closely related *X. strumarium* as a sedative, aphrodisiac, for fevers, malaria and urinary disorders. Leaf extract with honey for fever and cough, pounded leaves for ulcers, root for hormonal issues and as a bitter tonic. Decoction with sugar for diarrhea and seed oil for rheumatism. Paste of burrs for wounds.[121] In China an extract from the root is used for ulcers; in Germany they use it for malarial fever and in Russia for hydrophobia.

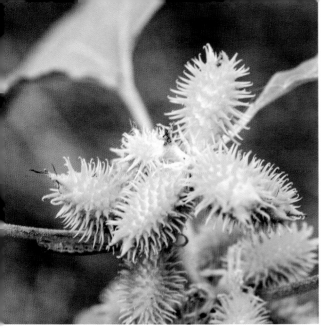
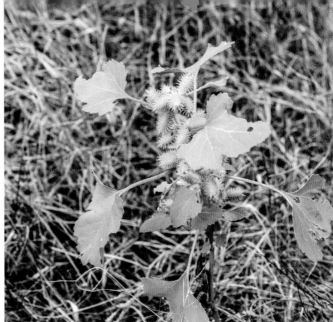

FARM/ENVIR. Noxious weed of summer crops such as cotton and sunflower. Contaminates stock feed and causes poisoning. Burrs adhere readily to livestock and clothing. Contamination of wool is a substantial cost to the industry. Can cause death in pigs if they eat large amounts while rooting and grazing on seedlings. Seeds are the most poisonous part but rarely eaten because of their spiny capsule. Mature plants also rarely eaten because of their bitterness and rough texture. Some botanists question its toxicity, only being poisonous in specific seasons.[122] Indicates soil very low in calcium, phosphate and very high in potassium, magnesium, manganese, zinc and other minerals. Low humus and hard crust.[8]

MAY BE CONFUSED WITH Four species of Xanthium occur in Australia along with the distinctive Bathurst Burr (*X. spinosum*). Hunter Burr (*X. italicum*), which has less noticeably lobed leaves, and spines on the tip curve inward. South American Burr (*X. cavanillesii*), which has barely dissected leaves, more triangular in outline. Burrs more globular and densely spiny. Californian Burr (*X. orientale*) leaves a cross between types and burrs have stout inwardly-curved terminal spines (like buffalo horns). All have similar properties to *X. occidentale*. Hybridizing with the numerous subspecies is common.

FURTHER READING Xanthatin and xanthinosin from the burs of *Xanthium strumarium* L. as potential anticancer agents.[123] Hepatotoxic constituents and toxicological mechanism of *Xanthium strumarium* L. fruits.[124]

WARNING Beware if you have an allergy to the Asteraceae family. Can also cause contact dermatitis in susceptible humans. Prolonged use of significant doses can cause toxicity in humans. Young plants and seeds causes toxicity if eaten in large amounts by animals.

NUTGRASS

Purple Nutsedge

Cyperus rotundas

DISTRIBUTION Cosmopolitan weed of over 90 countries and widespread throughout Australia.

HABITAT Weed of cultivated crops, market gardens, orchards, wastelands, wetlands, swamps, home gardens and parklands.

DESCRIPTION

Colony forming perennial sedge with wiry rhizomes. In cooler climates, the plant will flower within seven weeks after emerging and produce tubers. Cycle repeats itself several times during growing season.

LEAVES Dark green, strap-like leaves emerging at ground level and tapering to a point.

FLOWERS Loose umbrella-like tops of brown to purple.

FRUIT/SEED Seeds rarely viable, reproduction mostly occurs from the purple, round tubers or nuts growing in a chain of two to six on a rhizome.

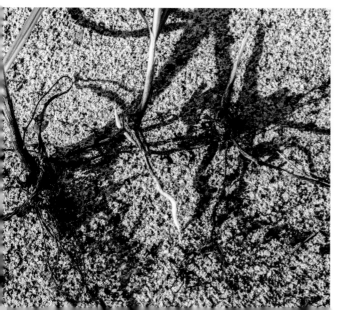
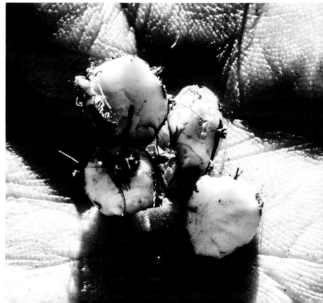

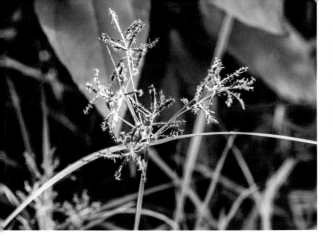
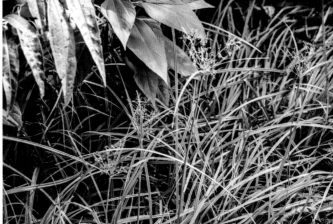

USES

EDIBLE/OTHER Nuts may be eaten raw, boiled or roasted but has a distinct Vicks VapoRub flavor which lessens with drying. I have eaten them raw and in a curry – interesting flavor! Australian Aborigines would roast and eat the nuts in many parts of the continent. Yellow Nutsedge (*Cyperus esculentus*) with yellowish-green tops are much nicer with a hazelnut flavor. This plant is less widespread, in Australia mainly on north coast of Queensland, North America and Southern Africa.

MEDICINAL One of the most extensively researched and non-cultivated plants on this planet. Why? This is such a valuable plant used for antimicrobial, antibacterial, antispasmodic, antioxidant, antiplatelet and anticonvulsant activities. Other uses are constipation, digestive problems, increases milk supply, insect repellent, wound healing, malarial fever and typhoid fever. Let's be aware of its uses and think of this plant in a different context. Its essential oil, 0.5–0.9%, is used in insect repellent cream, soap and perfume making. Use crushed fresh or dried nuts or rhizome juice internally, or make a tea, tincture or dried and ground and used in capsules.

FARM/ENVIR. A widespread weed that encroaches on every environment, much disliked by gardeners and farmers alike. Difficult to eradicate. However, pigs, geese and poultry will eat the tubers. This plant has commercial opportunities. Dry weight/hectare of underground rhizomes and nuts two–four tonnes when grown naturally and if grown on fertilized land six tonnes/hectare after 20 weeks. Nutgrass is shade intolerant so you can suppress it by growing a close-crop canopy all year round. Reduce growth by using translucent plastic film. Tubers are vulnerable to drying and intense freezing.[125] Its presence indicates soil low in calcium and phosphate and high in potassium, magnesium and iron. Low in humus, bacteria and compacted soil.[8]

FURTHER READING The incredible benefits of Nagarmotha (*Cyperus rotundus*). Antimalarial, antispasmodic, antidiarrheal, anticonvulsant, antioxidant, antibacterial, antiplatelet, lipid lowering and wound healing.[126] Antidiabetic in rats.[127] In vitro antibacterial, antioxidant, cytotoxic.[128]

OYSTER PLANT

Bear's Breeches

Acanthus mollis

DISTRIBUTION Native to Italy and the Mediterranean region. Has spread worldwide with cultivation. Naturalized in south-eastern Australia, especially Tasmania.

HABITAT Escaped cultivation as an ornamental and amenity plant. Grows in gardens, forests and conservation areas.

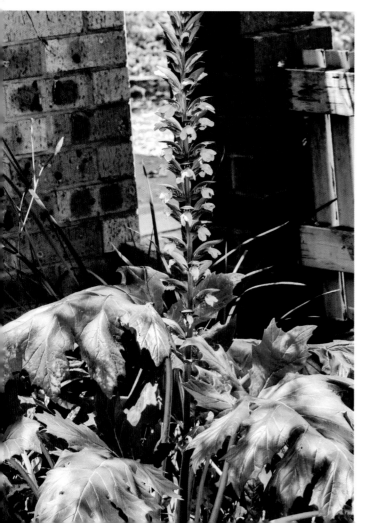

DESCRIPTION

Hardy, drought-resistant plant once established (two years). Clump forming perennial 1 m x 1 m (3 ft 3 in x 3 ft 3 in) or larger with strong rhizomes.

LEAVES Glossy, dark green leaves that are large and deeply lobed. Forms a basal foliage and dies down in cold areas.

FLOWERS Bold flower spikes are covered with 30 or more attractive flowers. They are creamy-white, like snap dragon flowers and each hooded with spiny reddish-purple bracts.

FRUIT/SEED Explosive pods scatter seeds over a wide area. Each seed capsule contains two to four large black seeds.

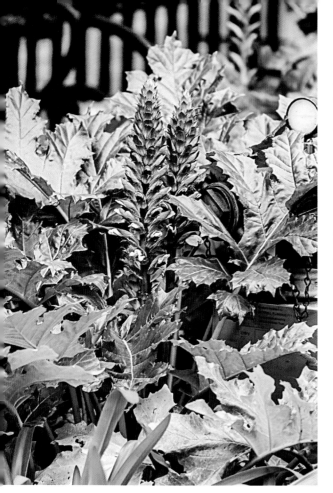
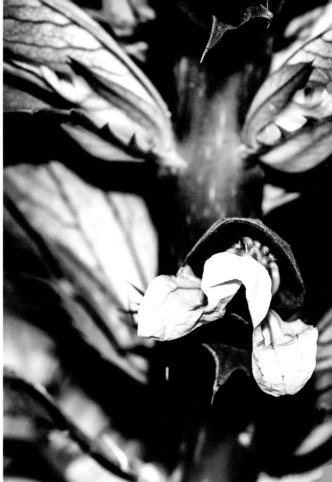

USES

EDIBLE/OTHER Not edible. A survivor from ancient Greece and Rome and the leaf copied as a motif on top of Corinthian columns.

MEDICAL A renowned medicinal herb in past years. Found in medicinal gardens in monasteries. Heals wounds, burns and used to treat dislocated joints. Internally soothes membranes in the digestive and urinary tracts. Crushed leaves used as poultices for burns, scalds and swollen legs. Used for digestive problems, diarrhea and clearing up phlegm.

FARM/ENVIR. Forms dense infestations under forest canopies and suppresses growth of natives. An environmental weed in Victoria and a potential threat to one or more vegetation formations. I always have a few plants in the garden for their beauty and their uses.

FURTHER READING Molluscicidal and cercaricidal efficacy of *Acanthus mollis* and its binary and tertiary combinations with *Solanum nigrum* and *Iris pseudacorus* against *Biomphalaria alexandrina*.[129]

WARNING Toxic if eaten in large amounts.

PADDY'S LUCERNE

Jelly Leaf, Indian Hemp, Arrowleaf Sida

Sida rhombifolia

DISTRIBUTION Cosmopolitan in tropics and subtropics. Naturalized in eastern and northern Australia.

HABITAT Widespread weed of pastures, gardens, roadsides and wasteland. Loves the higher rainfall areas.

DESCRIPTION

Robust, erect, perennial herb to small shrub with twiggy stems and deep taproot.

LEAVES Dull green, paler below, highly variable leaves, growing alternate on branches.

FLOWERS Pale yellow to yellow-orange, solitary or in clusters at end of branches or in forks of upper leaves. Flowers in the warmer months.

FRUIT/SEED Pods have fine irritating bristles that break into segments. Fruiting in the warmer months. Dies down in cooler areas in the winter.

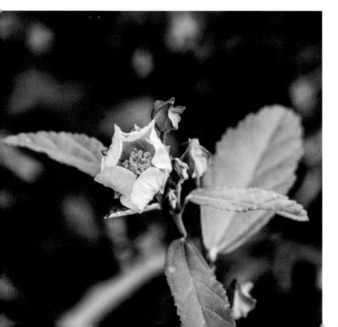
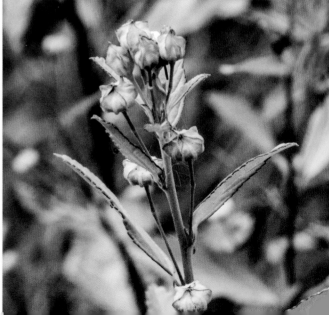

USES

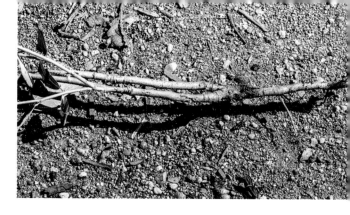

EDIBLE/OTHER Edible leaves and flowers, which also make a soothing tea. Stems used in making rough cordage, sacking and brooms. Stems have high quality fiber and once exported from India as 'hemp'.

MEDICINAL The *Sida* species are the most important medicinal plants in India. In Ayurvedic and Sidha medicine it is used for malaria, as an antibacterial, anti-inflammatory, antifungal, antispasmodic, for any problems with the urinary tract, sprains and rheumatism. Use the plant juice for headaches and flowers for wasp stings. Used crushed leaves for cuts, boils and wounds and boiled root bark for eczema. Root paste for menstrual disorders.[130] This plant is in the Malvalacea family so you can substitute it for any of the other mallows as it has high mucilage content especially in the stems. Thus good for protecting any inflammation and irritation of the throat. Relieves gastric ulcers, inflammation of the lungs and irritating coughs, bronchitis and TB. Australian aborigines used it to treat diarrhea and the leaves were a soothing smoke in Mexico. I make a cough syrup from the crushed roots, stems and leaves and it soothes the respiratory tract and brings relief to literally hundreds of people who have obtained the syrup from me.

FARM/ENVIR. Due to its high mucilage content, this is a great asset to any farmyard. Grow a patch for the animals to chew when they have diarrhea. Helps calves with white scours. Cattle and goats will generally eat this plant down to the ground, however horses do not like it. This plant is called 'Ironweed' because it's so difficult to pull up. Its deep taproot aerates the ground and brings up nutrients to replenish topsoil. However, this plant readily seeds and the plants can grow very thick and wipe out lower growing pastures. Stock will eat it without detriment but due to its fibrous nature it must be very indigestible and the ripe seeds of the plant are very irritating. Not the best fodder plant and difficult to eradicate. The ripe seeds have also caused the death of young fowls owing to their prickly character. Indicates soil low in calcium, phosphate, iron and sodium and very high in potassium. Low humus, bacteria, moisture and good drainage.[8]

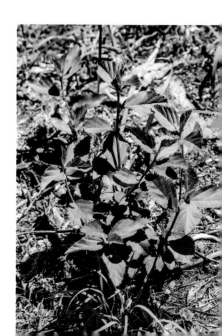

FURTHER READING Anti-inflammatory and antioxidant properties of *Sida rhombifolia* stems and roots in adjuvant induced arthritic rats.[131] Cytotoxicity and antibacterial activity of *Sida rhombifolia*.[132] Antiarthritic activity of various extracts of *Sida rhombifolia* aerial parts.[133]

PELLITORY

Pellitory of the Wall, Asthma Weed

Perictaria juduica

DISTRIBUTION Native of North Africa, Europe and Indian subcontinent. Now widespread in temperate and subtropical regions worldwide. Naturalized in southern and eastern Australia.

HABITAT Growing near urban areas, in walls, footpaths, embankments, cliffs, gardens and roadsides.

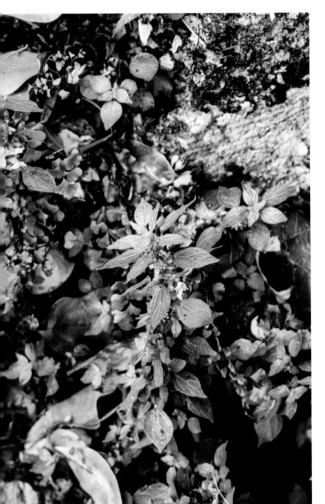

DESCRIPTION

Upright or spreading perennial plant, much branched, with hairy stems going woody and reddish-brown after it matures.

LEAVES Alternatively arranged, oval shaped, borne on short stems and covered in hairs.

FLOWERS Inconspicuous flowers borne in small dense clusters in leaf forks, initially green then reddish-brown as mature. Flowering spring to summer and warmer areas all year.

FRUIT/SEED Small, hard, dark brown/black.

USES

EDIBLE/OTHER Leaves and young shoots eaten in salads. Whole plant used to clean windows and copper containers.

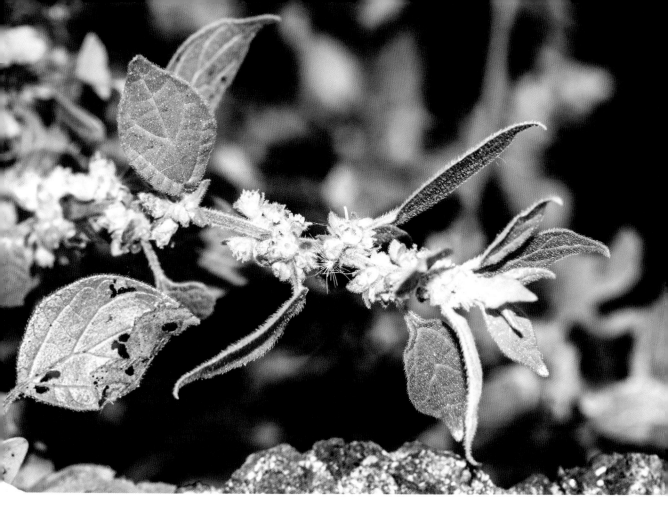

MEDICINAL Traditionally used as a tea, primarily as a urinary and kidney tonic. Current research has confirmed these uses. Used in the treatment of cough and sore throat as a decoction with honey. Other uses, hemorrhoids, gout, edema and recurrent cystitis.

FARM/ENVIR. Usually growing around cities and towns so not grazed by animals. Recently when I was in Sydney, I saw it growing out of numerous walls (as the name suggests). Often eradicated with herbicides, especially in the Sydney region where it is declared a noxious weed. Could be controlled better if everyone eradicated it by hand from their gardens.

MAY BE CONFUSED WITH Native Pellitory (*Perictaria debilis*) which is an annual with soft stems and smaller leaves on longer stalks.

FURTHER READING Good antiviral activity especially Herpes Zoster and feline immuno-deficiency virus (FIV).[134] Chronic kidney disease – nephroprotective.[135]

WARNING Sticky hairs on leaves may produce skin rash in sensitive people; pollen may trigger hayfever, conjunctivitis, rhinitis and asthma.

PENNYWORT

Indian Pennywort, Gotu Kola

Centella asiatica

DISTRIBUTION Native to the wetlands in Asia and now worldwide. Grows mainly along Australia's coastline and subcoastal areas.

HABITAT Widespread in damp ground, along roads, near swamps, in gardens, along water courses, woodlands and pastures.

DESCRIPTION

Perennial, low-lying herb with long, creeping runners, 2.5 m (8 ft) long. Rooting at the nodes with interconnection between plants.

LEAVES Circular or kidney-shaped with scalloped edges which rise above on reddish stems.

FLOWERS Small, inconspicuous flowers arranged in clusters, two to four flowers borne on stalks. Five pink, purplish or white petals with five deep purple stamens.

SEED/FRUIT Small fruits have seven to nine ribs and split when mature into two, one-sided segments full of tiny seeds.

USES

EDIBLE/OTHER Eating a few leaves a day is believed to help with arthritis and it makes a pleasant cup of tea. The Vietnamese serve Bai Bua Bok, a blended drink of Pennywort leaves sweetened with sugar and ginger.

MEDICINAL Due to ongoing research of this plant's healing and neurological properties it has become more popular. It restores and relaxes the nervous system; reduces inflammation (herb often sold as the arthritis plant); mouth ulcers, tuberculosis, fever, lupus, diabetic neuropathy, scleroderma and improves vigor and strength of the elderly. In India it is renowned for its use with leprosy and syphilis sores. In Indian folklore, there is a belief that this herb is the elixir of life, preserving brain, body and prolonging life. A true tonic.

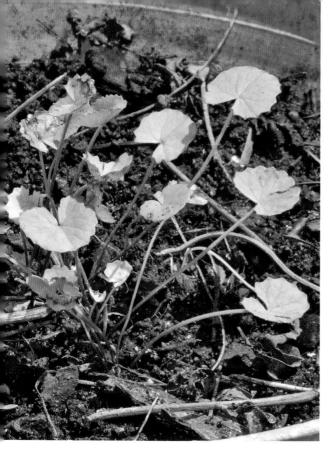
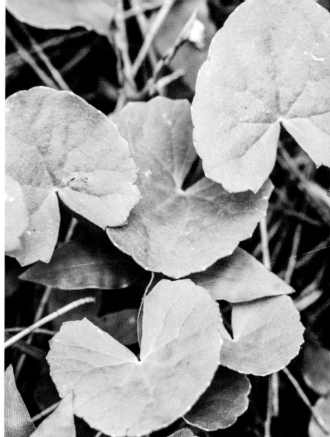

Externally it is useful for various skin problems, slow healing wounds, burns, ulcers, psoriasis, eczema, varicose ulcers, cellulite, after surgery and generally helps the small capillaries. I use the extract and tablets mainly to help concentration, relax the nervous system and as a tonic. I put the extract into a hydrating lotion I make as a skin treatment to help with cellulite, skin damage and general restoration of the tissue.

FARM/ENVIR. This plant has become naturalized all over the world and in countries such as America and Australia, subspecies have developed. The Pennywort that grows along my creek looks very similar but tastes milder than the one at my mother's place in Queensland. There needs to be more research and until its medicinal uses are proven, I will not use my local plant at my clinic but I will experiment on myself. It is a minor weed as not poisonous to stock and mainly grows in damp pockets. Indicates soil low in calcium, phosphate and high in magnesium with low humus and hard crust.[8]

MAY BE CONFUSED WITH Pennyweed (*Hydrocotyle tripartite*) which is native to Australia with inconspicuous greenish, yellow flowers. Found on the central coast of New South Wales, Queensland and Victoria.

FURTHER READING Pharmacological review on *Centella asiatica: A Potential Herbal Cure-all*.[136]

PEPPERCORN TREE

English, Chilean or Californian Pepper Tree

Schinus molle

DISTRIBUTION Native to South and Central America and introduced to warm temperate to tropical zones throughout the world. Naturalized throughout Australia.

HABITAT Escaped cultivation and naturalized in some areas. Pioneer species in its native range and elsewhere found in disturbed areas of secondary growth, roadsides, waterways and open woodlands.

DESCRIPTION

Evergreen tree 6–8 m (20–26 ft) high (occasionally growing to 15 m/50 ft) with weeping foliage. Trunk is short with deeply fissured bark. Fast growing.

LEAVES Long, narrow, hairless leaflets with variable margins growing alternately.

FLOWERS Drooping clusters of tiny, yellow flowers. Male and female flowers on different trees (female producing berries).

FRUIT/SEED Small, round, green berries that turn pink then black. One or two seeds/fruit. Seeds throughout the year.

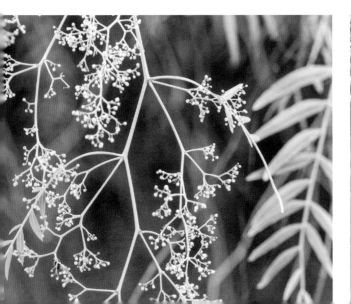
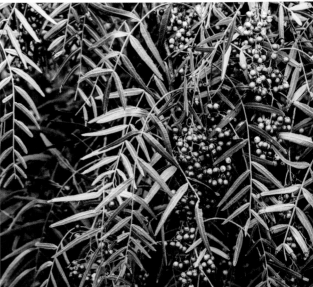

USES

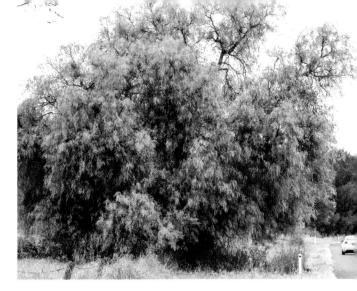

EDIBLE/OTHER Multipurpose tree commonly used in its native habitat by locals and harvested in the wild. Dried, roasted berries eaten as peppercorn substitute. Sweet, strong peppery taste. Intoxicating licorice and wines made from the fruit. Essential oil from fruit used as a spice in baked goods and sweets. Fruits pulverized and used in cooling drinks in South America. Gum used for chewing. Tannin from bark and an aromatic resin. Wood is resistant to white ants, durable, makes fence posts and used on the lathe. Wood is a good fuel and charcoal.

MEDICINAL Used for hundreds of years in South America. Rich in essential oils, new research backing up its traditional uses as an antiviral and antibacterial herb. Bark used as a tonic, to help hormonal and kidney problems and for skin problems. Useful for diarrhea, inflammation and tumors. Leaves used for rheumatism, as a stimulant and a calmer. Essential oil smells like fennel and pepper. Leaves are a good insect repellent and effective against common fungi.[137]

FARM/ENVIR. As a fast-growing, drought-resistant species it is useful in agroforestry. Planted for soil conservation, soil improver, windbreaks, shade and ornamental. Can grow on poor sandy sites in hot, dry positions and tolerates salinity. However, in some areas it is an environmental weed. On an old dairy farm where I lived once the cattle used to love camping under the shady peppercorn trees, planted for that purpose. People dislike them as white ants make their nests in the trees and they think they're an untidy, messy tree. That mess is good fertilizer for the topsoil and if you can easily locate a white ant's nest you can eradicate it.

MAY BE CONFUSED WITH Broadleaf or Brazilian pepper tree (*S. terebinthifolius*) which has spreading leaves with larger, broader leaflets.

FURTHER READING Chemical composition and anticancer and antioxidant activities of *Schinus molle* L. and *Schinus terebinthifolius* Raddi berries essential oils.[138] Chemical composition, insecticidal and insect repellent activity of *Schinus molle* L. leaf and fruit essential oils against *Trogoderma granarium* and *Tribolium castaneum*.[139]

WARNING Seed has an allergenic substance that can irritate mucus membranes. In large quantities toxic. Gum-resin and leaves can cause dermatitis on sensitive individuals. Pollen may cause asthmatic reactions.

PERIWINKLE

Blue Periwinkle, Greater Periwinkle

Vinca major

DISTRIBUTION Native to southern Europe and North Africa now widespread in Mediterranean climates. Naturalized throughout Australia.

HABITAT Garden plant that has escaped cultivation being found in gardens, urban bushland, open woodlands, watercourses, roadsides and waste areas.

DESCRIPTION

Perennial low growing plant with creeping or trailing stems up to 1 m (3 ft 3 in) long which may root at the tips. Hairless stems with milky sap.

LEAVES Paired, glossy, oval, green leaves.

FLOWERS Five petals, bluish-purple, tubular flowers borne singly in upper leaf forks. Flowers mainly in spring.

FRUIT/SEED Elongated fruit borne in pairs. Rarely seeds.

USES

EDIBLE/OTHER Not edible.

MEDICINAL Used mainly as a tonic and astringent internally and externally especially for excess menstrual flow, the urinary system, colitis, diarrhea, any excess fluid and blood. Chew leaves for bleeding noses and gums and for mouth ulcers. Also used for diabetes, hysteria, hypertension and tumors. Often used as a syrup. Made into ointment for piles and inflammatory skin problems. Contains alkaloids, the most useful being Vincamine, which is now mostly produced through semi-synthetic means.

FARM/ENVIR. It makes an excellent ground cover and I remember seeing it around the castles when I visited England. Can form dense, intertwined mats and cover large areas of woodland crowding out pasture. It is an understory species and prevents over-story species

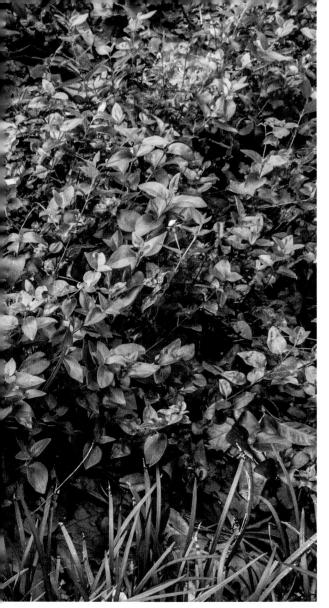
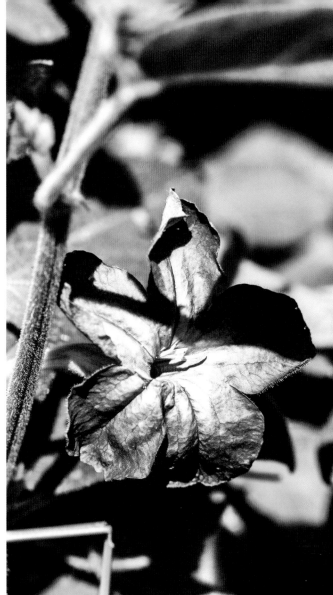

from growing. Avoid feeding animals on areas where there is an abundance of this herb as in large amounts it is toxic.

MAY BE CONFUSED WITH Lesser Periwinkle (*V. minor*) which has smaller leaves, stems and flowers. Used in homeopathy. Madagascar Periwinkle (*V. rosea* now *Catharanthus roseus*) more upright with pink or white flowers. Contains stronger alkaloids.

FURTHER READING Antidiabetic screening and scoring of 11 plants traditionally used in South Africa.[140]

WARNING Contact dermatitis with sensitive individuals. Contains alkaloids so use in moderation. It is toxic to horses, cattle and sheep if eaten in excess.

PETTY SPURGE

Radium Weed, Cancer Weed, Milk Weed

Euphorbia peplus

DISTRIBUTION Native to Europe, North Africa and Western Asia. Now growing worldwide in temperate and subtropical areas. Naturalized in southern and eastern Australia.

HABITAT Grows in gardens, footpaths, crops and waste areas.

DESCRIPTION

Annual plant, 5–30 cm (2–12 in) tall. Smooth and hairless stems which are green when younger and get a red tinge as mature. Recognized by the milky latex that oozes from broken stems and leaves.

LEAVES Soft, pale green with lower leaves stalked and alternate and upper leaves stalkless and opposite.

FLOWERS Small, umbrella-like structures are forked with minute, greenish flowers.

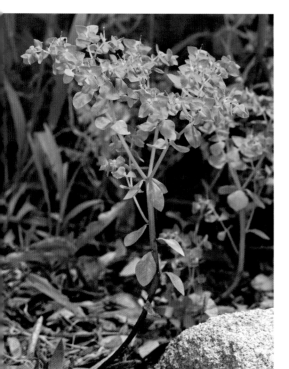

FRUIT/SEED Flowers are actually a cluster of small, leaf-like parts around a small, rounded seed pod which contains numerous seeds.

USES

EDIBLE/OTHER Do not eat this plant. Can be mistaken for Chickweed (*Stellaria media*) in its early growth and may be accidentally picked together for a salad. Your burning mouth (usually only symptom) will reveal your mistake.

MEDICINAL The sap has a caustic action, which is toxic to rapidly replicating human tissue. It is renowned for its use on suspect sunspots – those

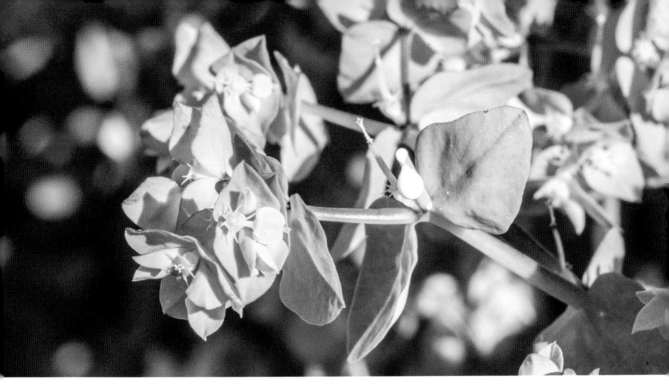

rough, raised lumps. In fact, 'physicians of the highest standing' would treat rodent ulcers (sun cancers) with this herb. In the *Medical Journal of Australia* in 1976 (Vol 1 page 928) a dermatologist wrote about its effectiveness. He advised to apply the latex daily for five days to remove basal cell carcinomas and it would leave no evidence of residual scar. For over twenty years I have been making an ointment from this and other herbs and in the last five years I have been making a cream using the juice of freshly picked plants which I preserve in alcohol. The latter has been the most effective. Today a patent has been taken out on the intellectual property surrounding the use of its active constituents and a pharmaceutical grade of gel has been approved by the US Food and Drug Administration for treatment of actinic keratosis (forerunner to basal cell carcinoma and squamous cell carcinoma).[141]

FARM/ENVIR. Environmental weed easily eradicated by hand pulling before it seeds. Always wear gloves due to the caustic action of the latex. Animals will usually avoid this plant due to its burning taste. Indicates soil very low in calcium and phosphate and very high in magnesium and potassium plus other minerals. Low humus.[8]

MAY BE CONFUSED WITH Chickweed (*Stellaria media*) which does not have white sap and trails along the ground.

FURTHER READING The sap from *Euphorbia peplus* is effective against human non-melanoma skin cancers.[142]

WARNING Toxic to humans and animals. Must be applied directly to the suspect sunspot, avoiding surrounding skin.

PLANTAIN

Narrow Leafed Ribwort, Greater or Broad Leaved Plantain

Plantago lanceolata, Plantago major

DISTRIBUTION Native to Europe and Central Asia and now growing worldwide. Ribwort naturalized in southern and eastern Australia and Greater Plantain grows on the east and south coasts and sub-coastal areas including Tasmania.

HABITAT Called 'White man's foot' it has followed white man wherever he went. Ribwort is found in pastures, cultivation, lawns, roadsides and wasteland. Greater plantain tends to grow in lawns, alongside drains, wherever the soil is damp.

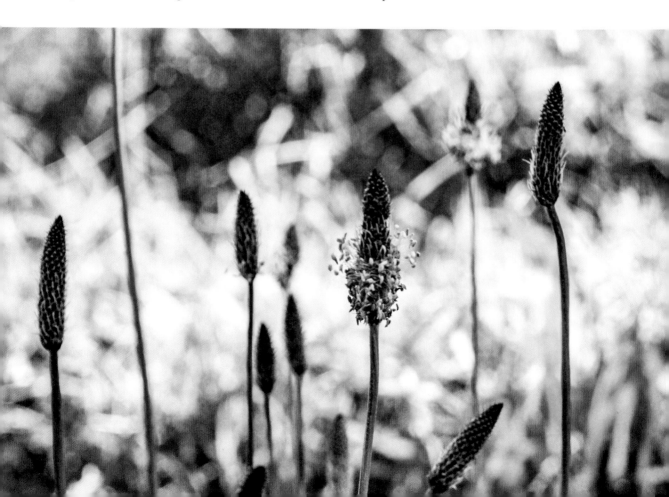

DESCRIPTION

Both plantains have a short, perennial rootstock, which sends up a rosette of leaves and flowering stems.

LEAVES Ribwort has lance like leaves, which may broaden in spring with three to seven distinct, parallel veins. Greater plantain has spoon shaped leaves with three to nine distinct, parallel veins.

FLOWERS Ribwort's long stem is topped with a cylindrical flowering spike 1–7 cm (0.4–2.8 in) long. Greater Plantain has inconspicuous flowers along the length of the stalk 5–40 cm (2–16 in) long. Will flower all year round but mainly in the warmer months.

SEEDS Tiny seeds which are high in mucilage and when wet stick to legs of passing animals. A healthy plant can produce 14,000 seeds per annum.

USES

EDIBLE/OTHER Leaves are edible but avoid older leaves, which are too fibrous. I use them more in juices and teas. The seeds are winnowed then sifted to get rid of the papery husks. You can use these in your cereal, bread or make a jelly-like tea. Psyllium husks sold in shops

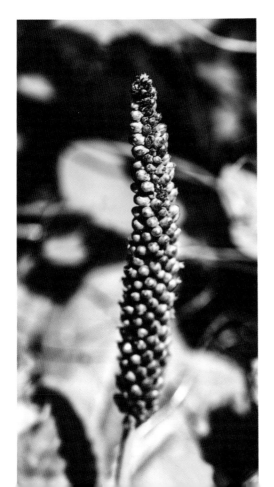
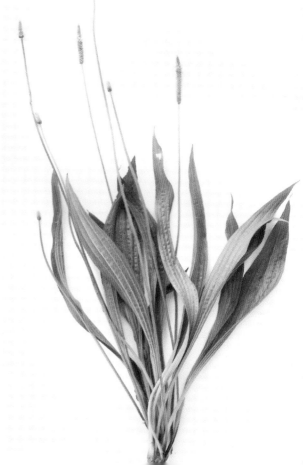

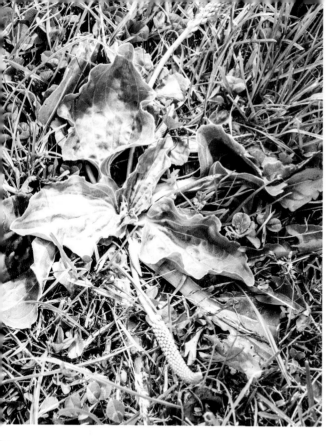
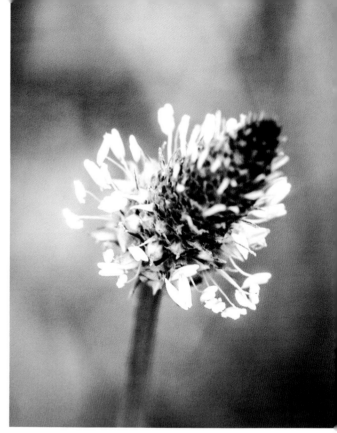
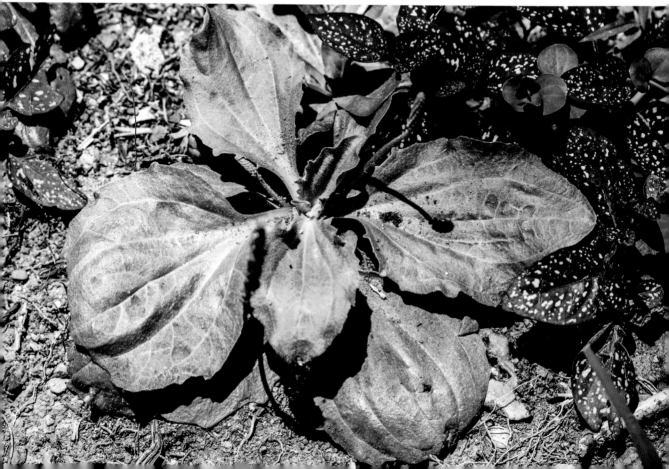

are from a cultivated species of plantain but you can use Plantain seeds as a substitute. An excellent, water-soluble fiber to help bowels. Seeds were found in Danish Peat bogs in the stomachs of ancient man.

MEDICINAL Used for centuries worldwide for many ailments. The main ones are for the respiratory system where it helps dry and nervous coughs, mild bronchitis, whooping cough, bronchial asthma, excessive phlegm, hayfever and sore throats. For the eyes use as an eyewash for conjunctivitis and inflammation of the eyelids. The kidneys as a diuretic, for cystitis, thrush and weakness of the bladder. The digestive system where it helps the bowels, hemorrhoids, diarrhea and constipation. This plant is known as 'ointment weed' as it is used as a poultice directly on the wound and can heal wounds, sores or ulcers even when nine years or more old. Research shows that the herb inhibits bacterial action and has anti-inflammatory properties. Used externally to give relief to stings and bites. It is an ingredient in my Cure-all weed ointment. This herb is a good tonic, enriches the blood and improves the lymphatic system. I use it as a tincture as well as a tea and a capsule.

FARM/ENVIR. Due to the ability of these plants to propagate readily and for their rosettes to compete with other vegetation they are rated as some of the most noxious worldwide weeds. In recent times farmers have been encouraged to grow a particular Ribwort in their pastures. *P. lanceolata ceres* tonic has been selected for pastures because it has a very high mineral count. Previously, in the UK farmers considered Ribwort a favorite food of sheep. Monoculture has its limitations and by bringing diversity to your farm the health of the animals will improve; I have introduced both Ribwort and Greater Plantain to our property. I started them in the garden and they soon left its confines to find their own niche. Wherever man has cultivated the soil, especially areas that have been trodden down such as in lawns and roadsides, up comes Plantain. If you wish to diminish its growth use fertilizer and sow Clover. The Plantain extract is used on stock for an antiseptic dressing. Indicates soil high in calcium, phosphate, potassium, magnesium and other minerals. Low humus, bacteria and moisture with hardpan.[8]

MAY BE CONFUSED WITH Buck's Thorn Plantain (*P. coronopus*) which has very variable leaves but they are lobed, and one to three distinct veins. Also more prostrate and has medicinal properties.

FURTHER READING Plantain (*Plantago lanceolate*) – a potential pasture species.[143] The traditional uses, chemical constituents and biological activities of *Plantago major* L. A review.[144] Antimony accumulation in *Achillea ageratum, Plantago lanceolate*.[145]

POPPY SMALLFLOWER OPIUM

Common Garden Poppy, Wild Poppy

Papaver somniferum ssp. *setigerum*

DISTRIBUTION Native to Europe and Mediterranean regions now widespread. Naturalized in southern and eastern Australia.

HABITAT Grows on roadsides, disturbed sites and occasionally cultivated areas such as wheat crops and fallow land.

DESCRIPTION

Annual, bluish-green, fast growing, erect herb 1–1.5 m (3 ft 3 in–5 ft) tall. Forms a rosette before stalk appears, shallow roots.

LEAVES Blue-green frosted appearance when young and mature leaves are stem clasping, oval with toothed margins.

FLOWERS Four paper-like petals, pink to violet with purple blotches at their base. Flowers in spring.

FRUIT/SEED Hairless, globular capsule with seven or eight ray-like ridges on top. When mature, pores open and release small, dull, dark seeds.

USES

EDIBLE/OTHER Seeds eaten raw or cooked. I use them the same way as commercial poppy seeds, but you'll only be able to collect small amounts. Young leaves and flowers eaten raw or cooked, pick before flower buds open. Eat moderately. Seed oil is edible, has an almond flavor.

MEDICINAL Flowers contain small amounts of opiates. The highest quantity comes from the latex. Used for pain, to relieve spasms, coughing, also good for fevers, promotes menstrual discharge, an astringent, helps restful sleep and is a sedative. This plant is closely related to the commercial variety which is grown for its opiates, which come from the latex.

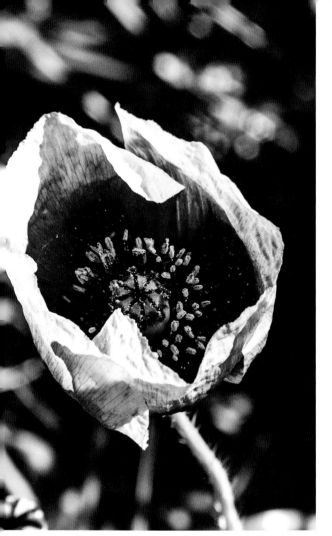
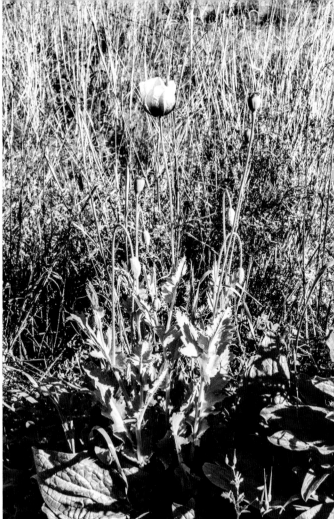

Commercially morphine, codeine and laudanum are made from this product.[146] This plant was on a list of medicinal plants in an Egyptian papyrus from 1,500 BC. I have trialed extracting latex from the small flowering poppy but it is very fiddly for little reward.

FARM/ENVIR. A minor weed and easy to pull up if needed. Seeding head is toxic to stock and poultry but they rarely eat it, and very few cases have been reported. In addition, the pain relieving effect is not as effective on animals as it is on humans. A pretty little plant appearing in spring.

MAY BE CONFUSED WITH Opium Poppy (*P. somniferum* ssp. *somniferum*) which has a much larger flower and fruit and greener leaves.

FURTHER READING Alkaloid content of *Papaver somniferum* subsp. *setigerum* from New Zealand (contains sedatives).[147]

WARNING Plant contains opiates. Toxic if seed heads eaten in large amounts.

POTATO WEED

Yellow Weed, Gallant Soldier

Galinsoga parviflora

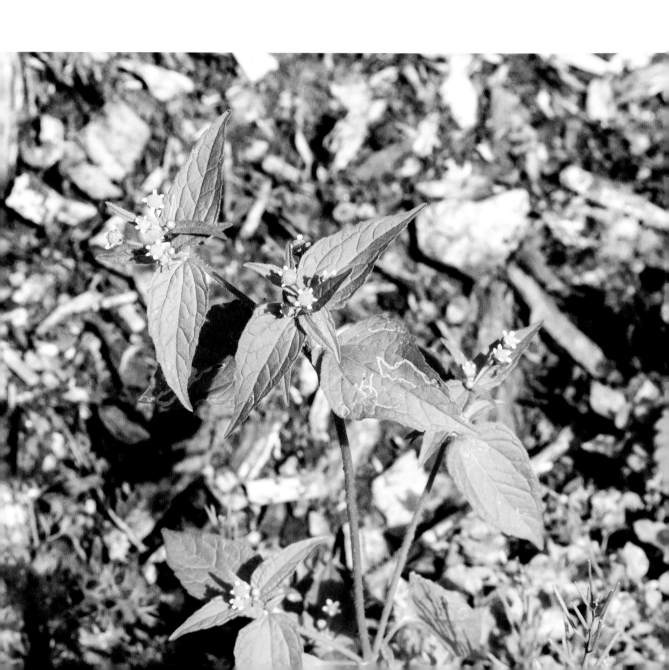

DISTRIBUTION Native of South America and now worldwide. Grows mainly along the Australian coastline and sub-coastal areas.

HABITAT A versatile weed, which requires moisture but will grow in any soil type or position. Found in cultivated beds, waste places and pavements.

DESCRIPTION

Annual, erect herb 20–70 cm (8–28 in) high, much branched. It has slender stems and shallow, fibrous roots. Plant has a short life cycle.

LEAVES Opposite, pale green, oval with a fringe of short hairs on the leaf margins.

FLOWERS Heads of numerous, yellow, tubular flowers with four or five white, three-lobed, small, ray florets that are separate from each other. Flowers from spring to autumn.

FRUIT/SEED Small, flat and black.

USES

EDIBLE/OTHER Leaves, stem and flowering shoots eaten raw or cooked. It has a hint of an aromatic flavor; a good addition to your salad. High in nutrients, a good addition to your next juice or smoothie. In Columbia they make a Bogota chicken and potato stew/soup which must have this essential ingredient added. When harvesting their crops they will first pick this herb to use in their cooking or dry it for later use.

MEDICINAL Use the plant juice to relieve nettle stings. A good astringent so it helps coagulate blood of fresh cuts and wounds. Also a good antioxidant.

FARM/ENVIR. Invasive weed in crops, as it is highly competitive and can spread quickly. Causes loss in yields and seed production. Control by manual pulling, crop rotation, mulching and biological means. Stock will eat it so not a problem in pastures. Research shows this plant strongly accumulates cadmium from contaminated soils.[149] Indicates soil low in calcium, high in potassium and magnesium with poor humus and bacteria. High moisture, poor drainage and a hardpan.[8]

FURTHER READING Distribution, biology, and agricultural importance of *Galinsoga parviflora* (Asteraceae).[148] Screening of a new cadmium hyperaccumulator, *Galinsoga parviflora*.[149]

PRICKLY LETTUCE

Compass Plant, Wild Lettuce, Wild Opium

Lactuca serriola

DISTRIBUTION Native to North Africa, Europe, India, western and central Asia. Grows worldwide and naturalized throughout Australia.

HABITAT Weed of agriculture, habitation, watercourses, disturbed bushland and National Parks.

DESCRIPTION

Looks like a prickly garden lettuce gone to seed. Tall annual, up to 2 m (6 ft 7 in), that starts with a rosette of leaves and grows a prickly stem with white latex. The stem commonly twists at the base to lie in a vertical plane, leaves point north and south. Grows in the cooler months.

LEAVES Broadly oblong, spiny along the margins and the lower rib. Stem leaves are alternate, dissecting and clasping the stem.

FLOWERS Numerous small, yellow flower heads in open clusters.

FRUIT/SEED From the small, white pappus yellowish-grey seeds fly away on small parachutes.

USES

EDIBLE/OTHER Edible young, tender leaves, raw or cooked. Eat in salads but bitter and more bristly as gets older. I chop the leaves finely and fry them in butter and even nicer with bacon. It may cause digestive upsets if eaten in large amounts. Some authors believe our common lettuces originally came from this plant.

MEDICINAL Latex contains lactucarium which helps to relieve spasms and pain, aids digestion, slows down urination, is a hypnotic and sedative. Like a mild opium. Not addictive. May help insomnia, anxiety, neuroses, hyperactive kids, dry coughs, whooping cough and rheumatic pains. Externally use the latex on warts. Best to collect the latex when

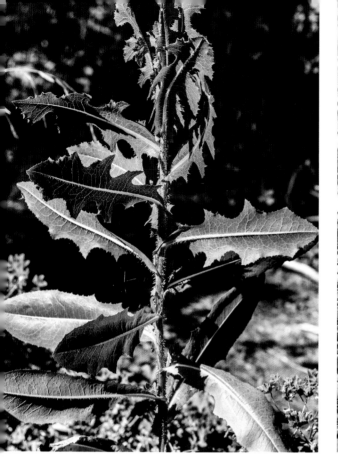
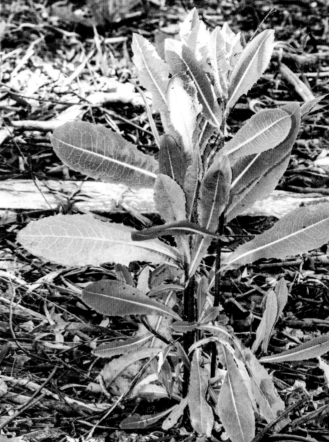

flowering. I cut off the top of the bigger plants and a large ball of latex oozes out of the stem. This will dry into a hard, rubbery ball, which is easily rolled off. Allow to dry longer in the sun and then store. Use one ball in a cup of boiling water and take as needed. It is extremely bitter and unpleasant to drink although it makes you feel at ease. One of my students told me she ate two leaves every morning and was relaxed for the rest of the day.

FARM/ENVIR. Environmental and invasive weed in native vegetation as it poses a threat to one or more vegetation formations. This plant is an effective soil builder. Its long taproot brings nutrients to the surface of the soil. When plants are mature or dry, safe for animals. Avoid stock grazing on large amounts of young plants. Indicates soil very low in calcium and very high in potassium, magnesium and high in manganese and iron. Low humus, bacteria, moisture and hardpan.[8]

MAY BE CONFUSED WITH Willowleaf Lettuce (*L. saligna*) which has leaves with no bristles.

FURTHER READING Pharmacological effects of *Lactuca serriola* L. in experimental model of gastrointestinal, respiratory, and vascular ailments.[150]

WARNING Clinical suspicion of toxicity, eat in moderation. Cattle have developed pulmonary emphysema after eating large quantities of young plants.

PRICKLY PEAR

Common Prickly Pear, Spiny or Common Pest Pear

Opuntia stricta

DISTRIBUTION Native of America and now widespread including throughout Australia, Asia, Middle East, Spain and Africa.

HABITAT Commonly found in paddocks, open woodlands and roadsides. I find them on the top of rock formations in the National Park. Wherever the birds have dropped a seed.

DESCRIPTION

Perennial cactus 1–2 m (3–6 ft 6 in) high.

LEAVES The green, fleshy pads are flattened, leafless stems, which are covered in small raised structures which bear tiny, spiny bristles. These may have no spines or one or two sharp spines 2–4 cm (0.8–1.6 in) long.

FLOWERS Large, solitary, pale yellow.

FRUIT/SEED Pear shaped, purple to red, covered in tufts of irritating hairs. Contains numerous, hard seeds. Ripen in autumn.

USES

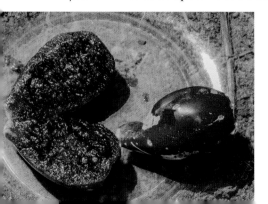

EDIBLE/OTHER Edible fruits, one of my favorites. Use gloves and/or tongs to carefully pick the fruit when about to fall or gather from the ground. Slice open and scoop out the tasty, slimy, purple flesh, spitting out the hard seeds. If you want to freeze or process them you will have to scrape off the irritating hairs in rough sand, using the bark of a tree, or use a scouring pad. Prickly Pear pads (see Leaves) are also edible but they have large spikes as well as hairs, which you must remove with the skins. Then eat raw in a salad or use cooked. If you do not like its slimy nature, you will have to boil for a short time in water with a pinch of bicarbonate of soda (baking

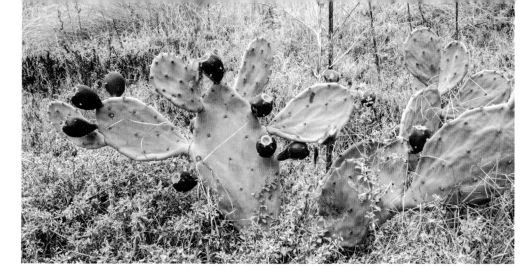

soda). Fruits make lovely sticky jellies, jams, candies and liquor. The pads were once a survival food of the American Indians and the hard seeds were ground to a flour. Other uses are the thorns used as gramophone needles and cochineal from the sap-sucking bugs that breed on various prickly pears.

MEDICINAL High in mucilage this herb protects the digestive tract, good for stomach ulcers, colitis, diarrhea and acute dysentery. I make a cough syrup from the fruits and find it is excellent for those difficult to heal coughs including whooping cough, asthma and other respiratory diseases. Externally poultices help inflammation, boils, wounds, chilblains and hematomas. In Mexico and other countries, it is used for diabetes. I have been experimenting with this on diabetics with amazing results. You soak clean pads, scour with a fork, cover in water and bicarbonate of soda and drink the next day.[151] However, the mixture is unpleasant, slimy and I had trouble getting people to take it.

FARM/ENVIR. Brought to Australia in the 1800s as a protective hedge and it spread at an alarming rate between 1870 and 1920. Australia's grazing land became so infested that the Prickly Pear Board was established and it was eventually biologically controlled with cactoblastis and cochineal insects. Although still widespread, it is no longer a major problem, most plants are infected by these insects. Some parts of the world still use it as livestock fodder. Once this plant is chopped down and dried, animals will readily eat it. Birds love the fruit. Indicates soil low in calcium, high in potassium with low humus, moisture and hard crust.[8]

MAY BE CONFUSED WITH Indian fig (*O. ficus-indica*) a tall 3 m (10 ft) garden escapee cultivated for its edible orange fruit.

FURTHER READING Diabetes is an inflammatory disease: evidence from traditional Chinese medicines.[152] Biological actions of *Opuntia* species.[153]

WARNING Injuries can occur from the small, irritating hairs and spines on the plant. I often get them on my tongue – most unpleasant.

PURSLANE

Pigweed, Wild Portulaca, Munyeroo

Portulaca oleracea

DISTRIBUTION Cosmopolitan and found throughout Australia.

HABITAT Rates amongst the world's most effective colonizing weeds, being native to most countries in the world. Growing wherever there is open, sunlit soil. Growing in gardens, pavement cracks, common weed of cultivation and wasteland.

DESCRIPTION

Annual, low-growing succulent herb appearing in the warmer months. Stems are juicy and often reddish-brown.

LEAVES Opposite, small and succulent.

FLOWERS Small, yellow, solitary or clustered growing in the fork between stem and leaf.

FRUIT/SEED Minute black seeds up to 10,000 seeds/plant.

USES

EDIBLE/OTHER High in vitamins A, C and E which are important antioxidants and many other nutrients including Omega 3 fatty acids – the richest source from a leafy green. The leaves and stems are eaten fresh in salads, use in juices, stir-fries, steamed or pickled. They taste like a slightly acidic Okra; a little slimy but this is good for your mucus membranes. Always use young leaves as oxalates increase as plant matures. Used for more than 2,000 years in India and Iran as a vegetable and eaten in most parts of the world. My favorite is Potato and Purslane Latkes, which you make like a fried potato cake or hash brown only you add chopped Purslane. You can also eat the tiny seeds, which you can collect in large numbers. The Australian Aborigines collected large quantities of the seeds, ground them and made them into cakes. When I tried this, my cake was very gritty; hard to keep out the dirt.

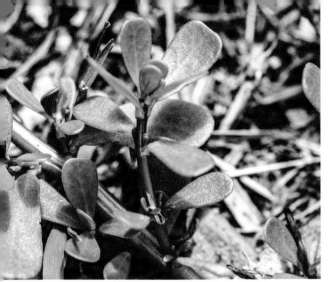
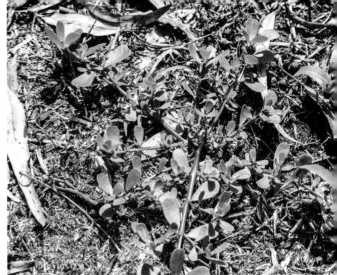

MEDICINAL Has numerous uses. Protects and soothes the whole urinary system and thus good for urinary infections and helps remove stone and gravel. Externally I use it like Chickweed (*Stellaria media*) as it is excellent for skin conditions especially the hot and itchy ones. I call it my 'summer chickweed'. Good for boils, ulcers, abscesses, eczema, burns and insect bites — use freshly crushed or as a poultice. For the digestive tract, helps with dysentery, bleeding, inflammation and liver troubles. For the respiratory system, useful for coughs and shortness of breath. Used in the reproductive system, for mastitis, increasing milk flow for nursing mothers. Also useful for inflamed eyes and low blood pressure.[154] I juice this plant and preserve it then add it to soothing creams.

FARM/ENVIR. As it produces a large number of seeds it will rapidly colonize any warm, moist site and become a solid carpet. If you do not remove all of the plant it will regrow after cultivation or tillage. Reduces aesthetic value of turf and ornamental plantings and can limit summer vegetable production. Reduce growth by growing strong competition, as it tends to grow on bare ground. Due to its high oxalate content never put stock on paddocks with high infestation of this plant. This year I have not been able to find any of these plants at our place as we've had a good season and good ground cover. However, I did find it trying to repair man-made damage. It was growing around trees that had a herbicide applied so that the ground was bare and hard. (In such cases these plants should not be eaten.) Indicates soil very low in calcium, phosphate and very high in potassium and magnesium plus iron and copper. Low in humus, bacteria, moisture and high in salt plus hard crust.[8]

FURTHER READING Common Purslane: a source of omega-3 fatty acids and antioxidants [155] Simple evaluation of the wound healing activity of a crude extract of *Portulaca oleracea* L.[156]

WARNING Contains oxalates. Suspected of causing nitrate and oxalate poisoning in stock.

RED FLOWERING MALLOW

Creeping Mallow

Modiola caroliniana

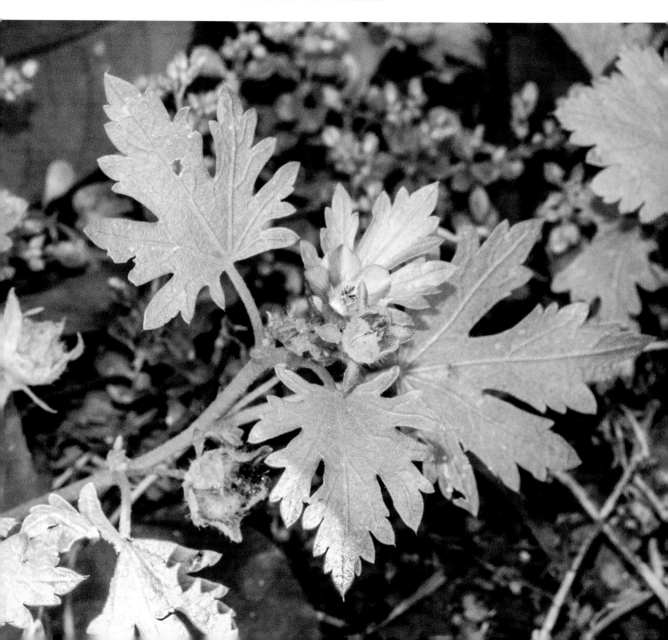

DISTRIBUTION Native to Americas. Now widespread throughout tropical and warmer temperate climates. Naturalized in southern and eastern Australia.

HABITAT Weed of gardens, lawns, footpaths, newly planted pastures and disturbed areas.

DESCRIPTION

A low-growing, creeping, perennial plant with long trailing stems that roots where the leaves grow (nodes).

LEAVES Single leaves arise from the stems that have an overall round shape with each lobe dissected into smaller lobes.

FLOWERS Five petals, small, orange-red flowers grow on long stems. Flowers mostly in summer.

FRUIT/SEED Wheel-like capsule made up of 20 black, hairy fruitlets. At maturity splits with two seeds/segments.

USES

EDIBLE/OTHER Contains toxins so not edible. Use as a medicinal tea.

MEDICINAL This plant is a member of the Mallow family (Malvaceae). Due to the presence of mucilage this herb is used for respiratory problems such as a dry, harsh cough, tonsillitis and a sore throat. Use as a gargle. It protects the urinary system, especially when inflamed, and has a soothing effect on the bowel. Can be used externally but I find Mallow and Paddy's Lucerne higher in mucilage.

FARM/ENVIR. Opportunistic and will grow anywhere there is cleared ground, even after herbicides have wiped out competition, it will keep growing. Always avoid using plants growing on land that has been sprayed. This plant has been suspected of poisoning and paralysis of sheep, goat and cattle so ensure you do not put stock in heavily infested paddocks. It is easy to pull out the whole plant if not wanted. I like the fact that it covers and protects bare ground.

MAY BE CONFUSED WITH Scarlet Pimpernel (*Anagallis arvensis*) which is also a trailing plant but has oval opposite leaves with red or blue flower.

FURTHER READING Hypotensive effect and enzyme inhibition activity of mapuche medicinal plant extracts.[157]

WARNING Toxic compound unknown but causes various problems of toxicity in animals. In other countries such as New Zealand research shows it is safe for animals so plant's toxicity must vary depending on soil and climate.

SAFFRON THISTLE

Saffron, Woolly Saffron

Carthamus lanatus

DISTRIBUTION Native to Mediterranean region and southern Europe. Spread to temperate parts of the world. Widely spread in central and southern Australia.

HABITAT Weed of crops, pastures, roadsides, rangelands and wasteland. Will tolerate very poor soils with low rainfall.

DESCRIPTION

Erect, spiny, annual herb growing 40–90 cm (16–35 in). Stems ribbed, profusely branched terminally and covered in minute hairs, often giving it a woolly look.

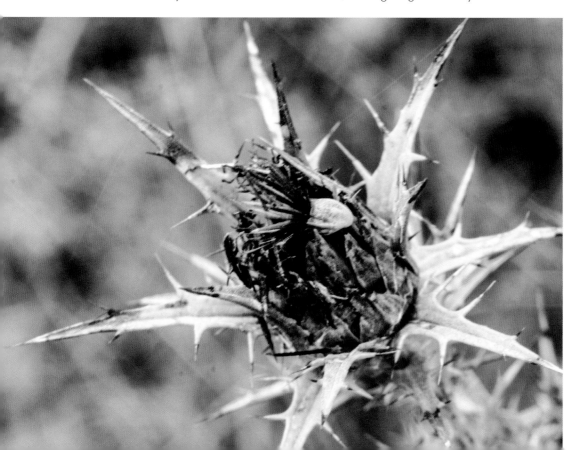

LEAVES Rigid, deeply-lobed, ending in a spine.

FLOWERS Yellow, surrounded by spines, flowering in summer/autumn.

FRUIT/SEED Single seed with rigid pappus, scales. Mature in autumn and may stay dormant up to eight years in soil.

USES

EDIBLE Rarely eaten but seeds high in oil and protein content.

MEDICINAL Closely related to Safflower (*C. tinctorius*) with its higher oil content and numerous medicinal qualities. Use the plant extract on the eyes for conjunctivitis.

FARM/ENVIR. Priority environmental weed in all states except Tasmania as it has inhabited natural habitats and conservation areas. An unpleasant thistle that can cover the property, contaminating hay and grain. The sharp thistles cause physical damage to stock especially causing eye infections and contaminating wool. Sheep, goats and birds will eat the seeds. Trials with a heavy population of goats resulted in excellent control (81%). My husband Bryant and I have spent many hours each year with the hoe on smaller infestations to eradicate it.

FURTHER READING Aerial parts anti-inflammatory and mildly analgesic.[158]

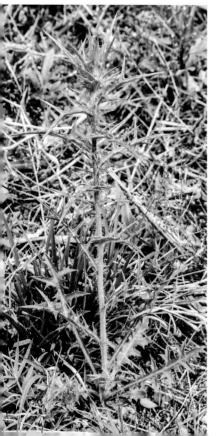
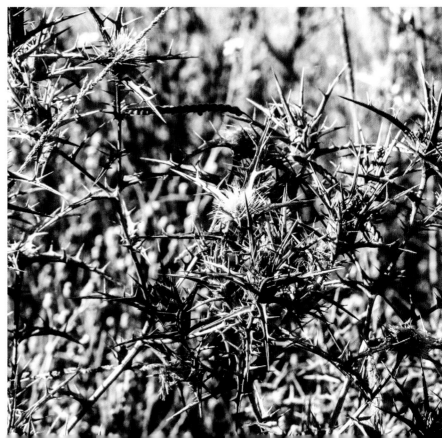

SALSIFY

Oyster Plant

Tragopogon porrifolius

DISTRIBUTION Native of Europe and North Africa and now spread to temperate regions. Naturalized in southern and eastern Australia.

HABITAT Found near habitation growing on roadsides, grasslands and wastelands.

DESCRIPTION

Erect, stout, short-lived perennial with an upright stem and a thick, fleshy taproot. Starts as a rosette and has white latex when damaged.

LEAVES Dull green, grass-like leaves that are stem-clasping.

FLOWERS Distinctive, lilac flowers on hollow stalks opening in the morning and closing in the day. Flowers in warmer months.

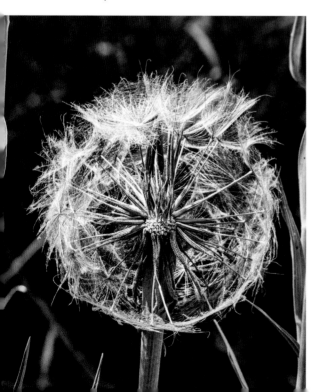
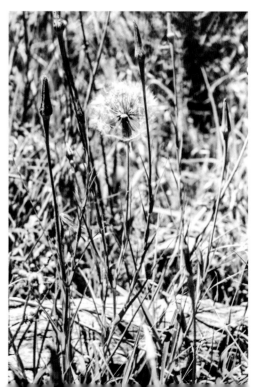

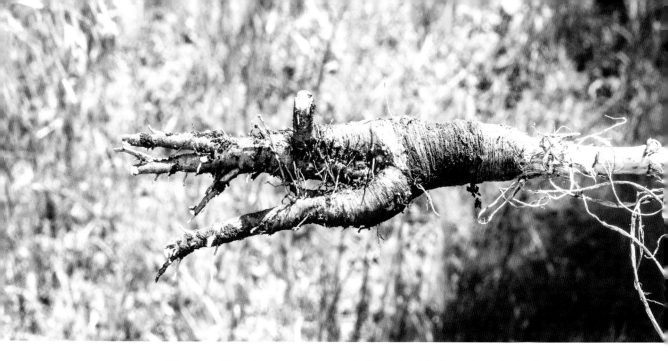

FRUIT/SEED Has a golden brown gossamer ball and ribbed seeds, which fly away on parachutes.

USES

EDIBLE/OTHER A popular root vegetable in eighteenth century. Britain and still cultivated in Europe and Russia. However, most people now grow the larger cultivated varieties. Edible leaves, shoots and roots. The root tasting rather like parsnips. Some authors say it should taste like oysters and occasionally you detect a slight seafood smell but I have never tasted a root that has a seafood flavor. You must dig up the knobbly root before the plant flowers, or it becomes very tough and fibrous. Cook just like parsnips. My favorite way is to roast the roots and grind to make a milo, or roast it more and create a coffee substitute. Very nice as a milky drink.

MEDICINAL Root is rich in inulin, a sweet, soluble fiber suitable for diabetics. Also an excellent prebiotic and helps digestion. Boil the root and make a decoction for liver troubles and loss of appetite.

FARM/ENVIR. An environmental weed in Australia and a priority weed in at least one natural resource management area. I often have problems finding good supplies as stock will graze on it. Best supplies around rivers and wasteland. Grows in full sun and likes dry conditions. It may be very difficult to dig up and breaks easily. Indicates soil low in calcium, high in magnesium, copper, zinc and selenium. Low in humus.[8]

FURTHER READING Bibenzyls and dihydroisocoumarins from white salsify (*Tragopogon porrifolius* subsp. *porrifolius*).[159]

SCARLET PIMPERNEL

Scarlet or Blue Pimpernel, Shepherd's Clock

Anagallis arvensis

DISTRIBUTION Native to Europe and temperate Asia now widespread in temperate regions of the world. Naturalized throughout Australia.

HABITAT Grows in lawns, garden beds, roadsides, pastures and wastelands.

DESCRIPTION

Low-growing, creeping, annual or occasionally perennial herb with square stems that branch from the base.

LEAVES Opposite and stalkless with shiny upper surfaces and underneath covered in minute dark hairs.

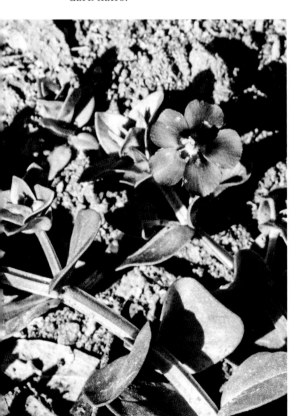

FLOWERS Single scarlet flowers with five pointed petals which grow on long stems. Alternatively, it may have single blue flowers. Some authors believe Blue Pimpernel is a subspecies and you often see them growing together. The flowers are sensitive and only open on bright days. Flowers mainly in spring.

FRUIT/SEED Small dark angular.

USES

EDIBLE/OTHER Not edible as contains toxins. Once a famous cosmetic herb regularly employed to fade those 'unsightly freckles'. I use this in my Ladies Bedstraw cream, which helps to fade spots, pigmentations and freckles.

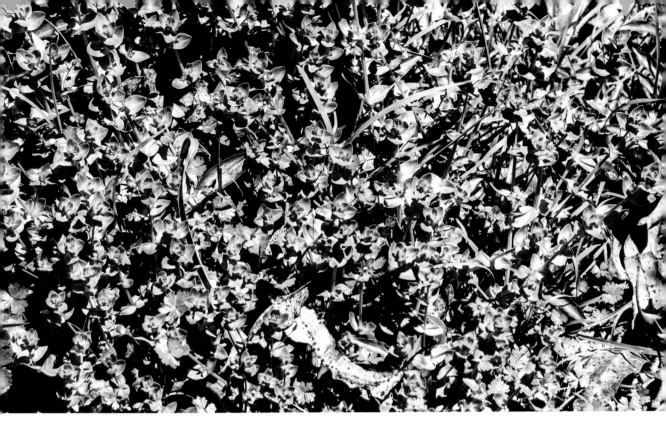

MEDICINAL Once a panacea for all ills. Used for melancholy and allied forms of mental illness. Many authenticated accounts of epilepsy being completely cured by it. I have trialed it on an epileptic dog with good results. Strongly antifungal, heals wounds, diseases of the eyes, especially for the dim-sighted, draws out thorns and splinters and used for rheumatism. Used to treat dropsy, gout, leprosy and helps move phlegm, a good kidney and fever herb.

FARM/ENVIR. If stock left in a heavily infested paddock they would get general depression, suspension of rumination, diarrhea and thirst. Incidence of toxicity in stock is rare and variable. This little ground cover plant threatens and endangers native species as it takes over their niche. It will cover bare ground quickly and compete with other young plants. On our property we have good ground cover so this plant only pops up here and there, mainly on bare or disturbed land. I love its vivid flowers and in general find a predominance of the red flowering variety on acidic soils and a predominance of blue flowering on alkaline soils. Indicates soil low in calcium and phosphate and low in humus and bacteria.[8]

FURTHER READING In vitro antiviral activity of a saponin from *Anagallis arvensis*, Primulaceae, against herpes simplex virus and poliovirus. Antiviral research.[160] Antifungal properties of *Anagallis arvensis* L.[161]

WARNING Narcotic so only have for medicinal purposes. Toxic in large amounts to stock.

SELF HEAL

All Heal, Heart of the Earth

Prunella vulgaris

DISTRIBUTION Cosmopolitan and naturalized in south-eastern Australia.

HABITAT Roadsides, paddocks, lawns, waste grounds, especially damp places.

DESCRIPTION

Low-growing, perennial, sparingly hairy. Creeps along the ground striking at the nodes.

LEAF Oval and slightly indented, green with a reddish-purple tinge.

FLOWERS The dense terminal spikes are made up of numerous bluish-purple flowers, hooded and lipped. Flowering in the warmer months.

FRUIT/SEED Smooth oval nutlets, two-celled with black seeds.

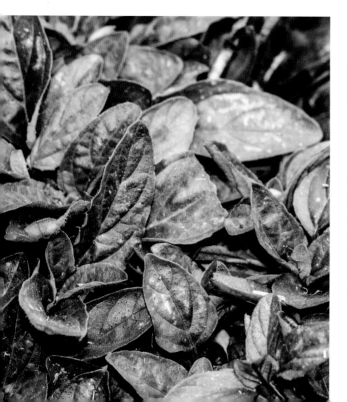

USES

EDIBLE/OTHER Used as a medicinal herb. Makes a soothing cup of tea but has a bitter flavor.

MEDICINAL Culpeper, a famous nineteenth century English herbalist, explained the name 'Self-Heal whereby when you are hurt, you may heal yourself'. An excellent antioxidant, anti-inflammatory and astringent. Useful to bring up phlegm, for a dry cough, sore throat, fevers, headaches, gum inflammation and conjunctivitis. Externally a good

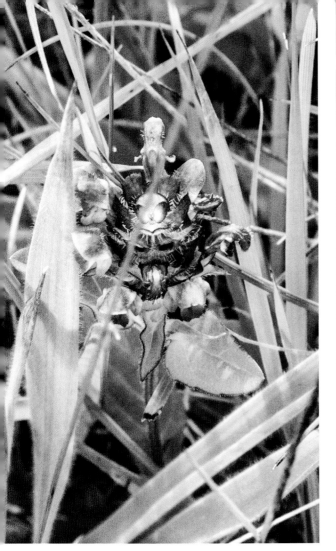
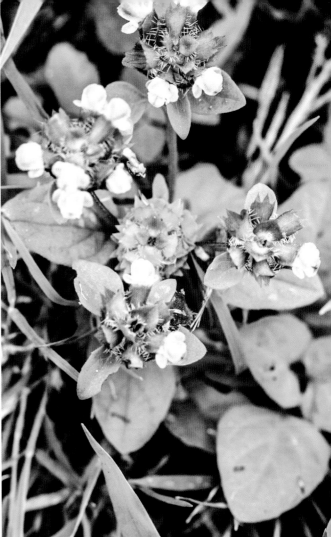

wound herb especially with excessive bleeding and useful for skin inflammation and boils.

FARM/ENVIR. Growing in cooler, damp soil it is mainly a problem in sub-alpine areas where it displaces native vegetation. It does not grow on my property unless I plant it and then it tends to die off in the hot summers. I have found a number of patches of this herb growing in damp, shady areas and in the cooler mountains nearby. In cooler areas and especially in Europe and North America it grows in abundance and often displaces native vegetation. Indicates soil low in calcium high in phosphate and very high in potassium, magnesium, manganese and other minerals including selenium. Low humus, poor drainage, high moisture and hardpan.[8]

FURTHER READING Anti-allergic and anti-inflammatory triterpenes from the herb of *Prunella vulgaris*.[162] Mechanism of inhibition of HIV-1 infection in vitro by purified extract of *Prunella vulgaris*.[163]

SHEEP SORREL

Field Sorrel, Sour-weed

Rumex acetosella/Acetosella vulgaris

DISTRIBUTION Native to western and central Europe, now growing throughout the world in temperate and subtropical areas. Naturalized in southern and eastern Australia.

HABITAT Growing in crops, pastures, gardens, footpaths, heathlands, wetlands and alpine areas.

DESCRIPTION

Perennial, small, clumping plant with extensive underground system of roots. Flowering stem 10–60 cm (4–24 in) tall.

LEAVES Distinctive arrowhead-shaped with two basal lobes.

FLOWERS Flower head made up of tiny reddish flowers on a slender stem. Male and female grow on separate plants. Flowering in spring.

FRUIT/SEED Tiny, three-sided, staying hidden in flower as it dies.

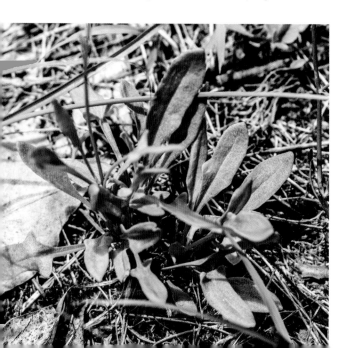

USES

EDIBLE/OTHER A tart lemony flavor, which I have found makes a tasty condiment and use it raw in a fish sauce. Loses its tartness if cooked. In Europe, eaten as a spring salad since time immemorial. This plant was held in great repute in Henry VIII's time but fell from favor when French Sorrel (*R. acetosa*) with its larger leaves was introduced.

MEDICINAL Good for vitamin C, fluid retention and cooling. Make a tea for fevers and it will quench the thirst. Once used for catarrh, hemorrhages, urinary disorders (avoid if you have gout due to the oxalates), as a gargle for ulcers in the mouth and used to heal wounds. Also used for toothache. The formula 'Essiac' created by Rene M Caisse RN in 1922 in Canada was to treat cancers. Its main ingredient was Sheep Sorrel, which was considered to be the main herb for tumors.[164] Many authors believe this herb to be anticancer, anti-inflammatory, antibacterial and antioxidant.

FARM/ENVIR. Environmental weed that invades native areas and displaces native plants. Creates dense carpets on bare ground in the alpine and other regions in Australia. Reduces grazing capacity. Not a major problem with stock as they dislike its taste. Weed of crops. Indicates soils very low in calcium and phosphate and high in potassium and magnesium. Low humus, sandy soil and presence of aluminum.[8]

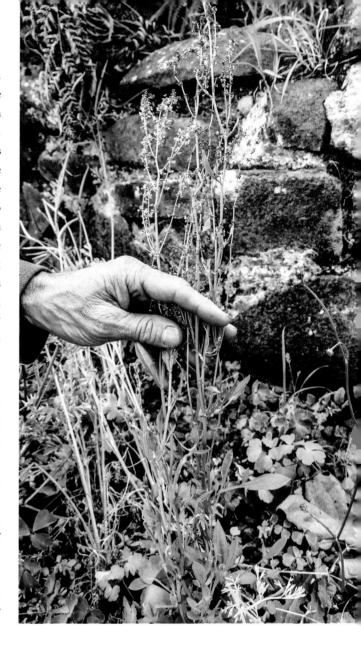

MAY BE CONFUSED WITH Rambling Dock (*Acetosa sagittata*) and Rosy Dock (*Acetosa vesicaria*). Sheep Sorrel distinguished by male and female on separate plants and fruit have no wings or teeth.

FURTHER READING Effects of sulphadimethoxine on cosmopolitan weeds (*Amaranthus retroflexus* L., *Plantago major* L. and *Rumex acetosella* L.[165]

WARNING Contains oxalate and nitrate.

SHEPHERD'S PURSE

Shepherd's Heart

Capsella bursa-pastoris

DISTRIBUTION Native to Europe and now cosmopolitan. Naturalized throughout Australia.

HABITAT Grows in gardens, disturbed habitats, lawns, pastures and crops.

DESCRIPTION

Annual, slender plant that starts with a rosette of leaves and stems grow from 3–70 cm (1.2–28 in) in height.

LEAVES Variously lobed with upper leaves clasping the upright spreading stems.

FLOWERS Tiny, white with four petals in loose clusters at the top of the stem. Flowers in the cooler months.

FRUIT/SEED You can recognize this plant by its heart-shaped fruits that are divided into two cells, containing numerous oblong, yellow seeds.

USES

EDIBLE/OTHER This herb is a member of the *Cruciferae* family (cabbage) and the leaves have a cabbage flavor. In China, they have bred a lush cultivated variety, sold in markets. In winter when there are fewer greens available this herb is a welcome addition to the diet. Chop the fresh leaves and use in a salad or in your juice. Leaves may also be cooked. I often pick the plant, just leaving enough so it can reshoot. The tops, especially the spicy seedpods are good eating. These minute seeds can also be roasted and eaten. The seeds were an ancient human food, deposits found dated to 5,800 BC.

MEDICINAL According to the 'doctrine of signatures' plant structure can indicate how they can be used. For instance, the heart-shaped seedpods tell you this plant is good for the circulatory system. Used as a tea it is still popular to stop hemorrhage or bleeding of all kinds. It regulates menstruation and corrects high and low blood pressure. It also helps

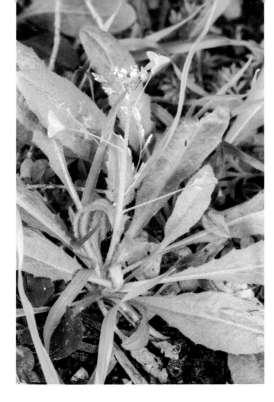
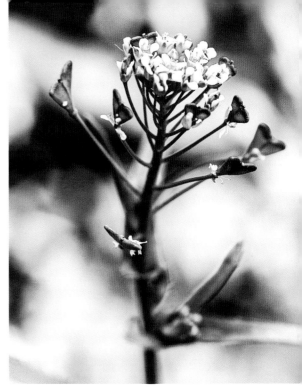

with kidney infections, water retention, kidney gravel and ulceration of the bladder. Effective for diarrhea. When the herb is dried or made into a tincture, it has a distinct yeasty smell. I use this herb as a tea, tincture or capsule especially for heavy menstruation. Nosebleeds are a common complaint and I have helped many people with this simple herb.

FARM/ENVIR. A serious environmental weed in most states in Australia. Displacing native vegetation and invading farmland. Rosettes cover the ground and little else can grow. Part of my lawn turns into a Shepherd's Purse plot in the winter months. Livestock will eat it and combined with cultivation this herb can be kept in control. For the wild birds in winter this dainty herb is a treasure as they love the seeds. However, it may turn your chook's egg yolks olive with a strong flavor. It can also taint cow's milk. In England the plants are made into a strong decoction and given to calves for diarrhea and purging. This herb absorbs excessive salts in the soil and returns them in their organic form. Research is also looking at using this plant as a biomarker for heavy metals.[166] Indicates soil very low in calcium, and very high in magnesium and other minerals. Low humus, low moisture, salty with good drainage and presence of aluminum.[8]

MAY BE CONFUSED WITH Penny Cress (*Thlaspi arvense*) which has edible leaves and seeds. Fruits flattened and more oval shaped with winged edges.

FURTHER READING *Capsella bursa-pastoris* L. Medic. as a biomonitor of heavy metals.[166] Inhibitory effect of *Capsella bursa-pastoris* extract on growth of Ehrlich solid tumor in mice.[167]

SLENDER CELERY

Marsh or Fir Leafed Celery

Apium leptophyllum

DISTRIBUTION Originated Central America now widespread including southern, central and eastern Australia.

HABITAT Winter weed of agriculture, creek banks, rainforest margins, gardens and shaded areas.

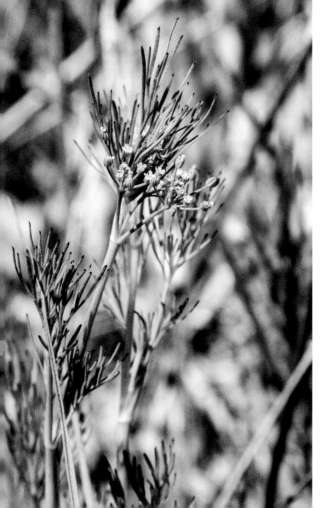

DESCRIPTION

Delicate annual weed up to 60 cm (24 in) tall related to celery, celeriac and sea celery.

LEAVES Shiny, thread-like leaves that have a feathery nature.

FLOWERS Clusters of tiny, white flowers on the end of a single stalk. Flowers in winter.

FRUIT/SEED Fruits are round/flattened, brown when ripe. Made of two fruitlets with five obvious ribs.

USES

EDIBLE/OTHER Has a distinct flavor reminiscent of parsley and celery. I think this plant should be grown as an edible herb not only for its flavor but also for the decorative leaves to garnish dishes.

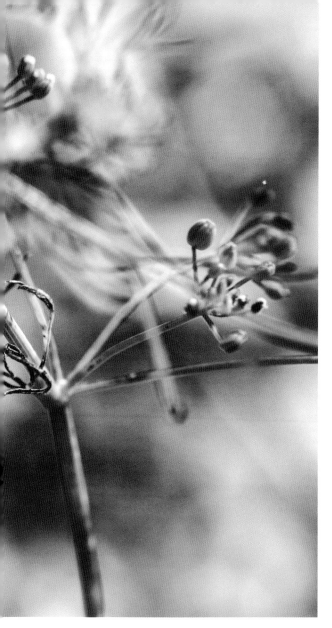
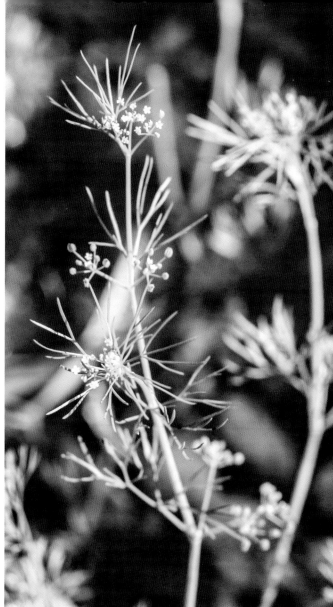

MEDICINAL Popular medicinal cultivated herb of India. In Ayurvedic medicine the dried fruits are collected by thrashing plants on a mat then drying the fruits. The essential oils are calming, antifungal, antibacterial and good for worming. Other uses, as a diuretic, sedative, for rheumatism, and for chronic skin conditions such as psoriasis.

FARM/ENVIR. Good fodder. Believed to taint milk but tests are inconclusive. Minor weed. I find this little plant growing all around habitation and in gardens. I pick it for my students and they are always surprised at its distinct taste.

FURTHER READING Chemopreventative potential against DMBA induced skin carcinogens.[168]

SOW THISTLE

Milk Thistle, Cocky Weed, Puha (Maori)

Sonchus oleraceus

DISTRIBUTION Native to Europe, North Africa and Asia and widespread throughout the world. Some botanists believe that it has been in Australia for thousands of years. Naturalized throughout Australia.

HABITAT Grows in garden beds, lawns, disturbed lands, pastures, crops, wasteland and roadsides.

DESCRIPTION

Erect, annual herb 0.5–1.5 m (1 ft 6 in–5 ft) tall that has a hollow stem that when cut exudes a milky sap. Short taproot. Differs from true thistles as they have flowers without a spiny base. Grows all year round.

LEAF Soft bluish-green leaves that clasp the stem. The leaf is deeply lobed with irregularly toothed margins ending in small, soft spines.

FLOWERS Bright yellow disc, 2 cm wide in a ray formation, like a small Dandelion flower.

FRUIT/SEED Small gossamer balls that house rough seeds with no beaks and that fly away on 'parachutes'. Grows all year round.

USES

EDIBLE/OTHER A tasty, crunchy weed that has a lettuce-like flavor. I love eating the small plants when young; they are just like little lettuces. I let the mature plants go to seed and encourage their growth. Full of nutrients, an excellent green in your salads, use the older plants for juices, stir-fry or other dishes, makes a pleasant tea.

MEDICINAL Being high in vitamins and minerals it makes an excellent tonic. Make a cup of tea and drink it when you have a fever. Other uses are the roots used as antibacterial and for worms; leaves are more calming so use as a sedative, for stomach problems, to help

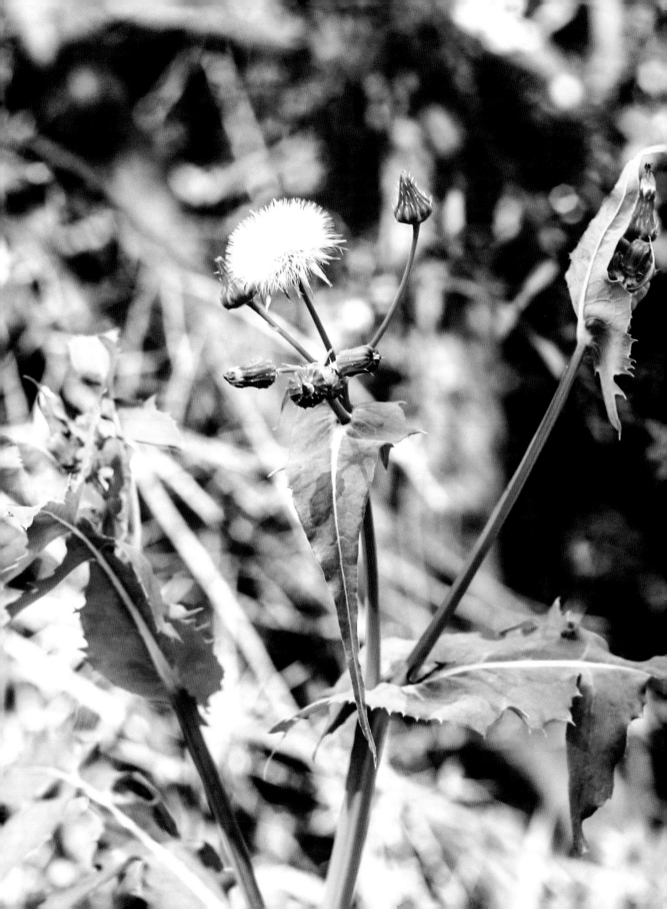

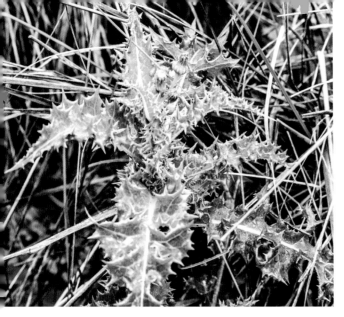
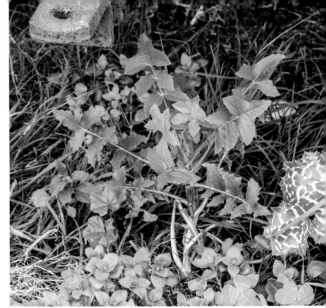
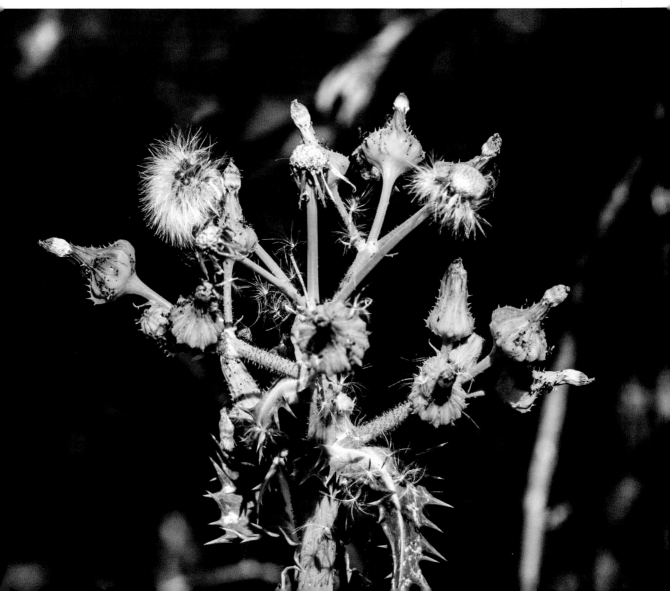

the liver and kidneys and for anemia. Also a specific for bronchial infections with yellow phlegm and an effective antioxidant. The brownish gum is used very effectively for liver, duodenal and colon problems but will cause griping. Keep to a minimum. Has many other uses from all over the world.[169] Externally it makes a calming balm for the skin. The white sap is used externally on warts.

FARM/ENVIR. Known as one of world's worst weeds, a pest in 55 countries, probably due to the prolific amount of seeds (25,000 seeds in a single plant) and their 90% germination. Problematic in grain growing areas where it reduces crop yield, interferes with harvest and contaminates grain. Problem in controlling this plant due to a combination of no-till farming and reliance on herbicides. Now some plants are herbicide resistant. Rabbits, hares, birds, poultry, pigs and cattle love eating this plant. Easy to pull up in the home garden but best to add it to your diet. Used for diarrhea and vaginal prolapse in stock. Indicates soil low in calcium, very low in phosphate, very high in potassium, magnesium and manganese plus other minerals. Good drainage and presence of aluminum.[8]

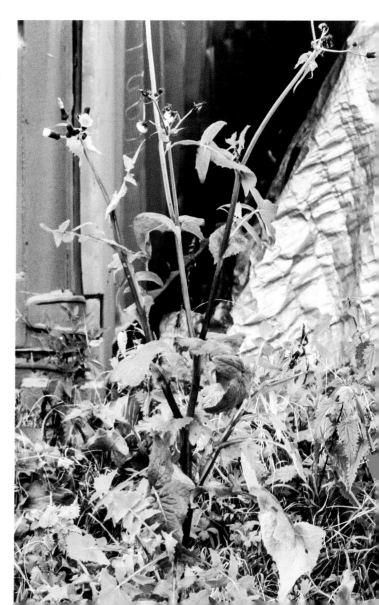

MAY BE CONFUSED WITH Prickly Sow Thistle (*S. asper*) and Native Sow Thistle (*S. hydrophilus*) are common, widespread weeds in Australia having stiff, leathery leaves with spinier margins. Seeds also vary.

FURTHER READING Nutritional composition of *Sonchus* species (*S. asper* L., *S. oleraceus* L. and *S. tenerrimus* L.).[170] Anxiolytic-like effect of *Sonchus oleraceus* L. in mice.[171]

WARNING Some authors stated that this herb is mildly toxic to animals if eaten in excess. There seems to be minor evidence to support this fact. Some authors believe it should be avoided if pregnant.

SPEEDWELL, CREEPING

Blue, Buxbaum's, Persian and Bird's eye Speedwell

Veronica persica

DISTRIBUTION Native of western Asia and now widespread in Europe, North America, North Africa, Japan, Australia and New Zealand. Naturalized mainly in south-eastern Australia.

HABITAT Commonly found in garden beds, lawns and also a weed of cultivation.

DESCRIPTION

Sprawling annual herb that roots at the nodes.

LEAVES Mid to dark green that are oval to heart shaped with scattered hairs. Margins are scalloped.

FLOWERS Solitary, pale blue with four rounded petals. Flowers have a white center and the petals have fine white lines running through them. Flowers spring and early summer.

FRUIT/SEED Capsule is net-patterned when dried with numerous flattened seeds.

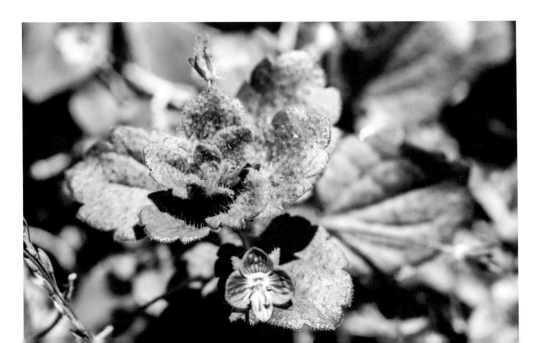

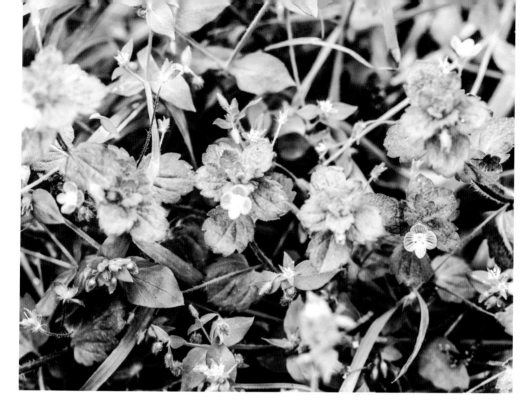

USES

EDIBLE/OTHER Eaten in salads, smoothies and cooked dishes however is bitter tasting and slightly hairy. I only eat it moderately but love using the little flowers to decorate food. Once used in 'tussie-mussie', a fragrant bouquet of flowers given as a farewell gift.

MEDICINAL Related to Common Speedwell (*V. officinalis*) and shares many of its uses. Gypsies used it as a 'blood purifier' and for the respiratory tract where there is a cough and excess mucus. Make the tea for sinus and for the eyes. I have trialed it to ease sore eyes and it does help. Relaxes muscles. Externally for skin rashes and inflammation.

FARM/ENVIR. This is a weed of 27 crops in 45 countries and may grow in grain crops. A main concern being that it is a host for a range of crop pests and pathogens. Easily diminished with dense crop population. I found this in my garden bed growing amongst my lettuces then noticed it all over the lawn. A pretty plant that covers the ground but very easy to pull up. Indicates soil low in calcium and phosphate and very high in potassium and magnesium. Low humus.[8]

MAY BE CONFUSED WITH Ground Ivy (*Glechoma hederacea*) also a trailing plant but it has clusters of three blue/violet flowers.

FURTHER READING In vitro cytotoxic activity and structure activity relationships of iridoid glucosides derived from *Veronica* species.[172] Phenylethanoid and iridoid glycosides from *Veronica persica*.[173]

SPINY EMEX

Cape Spinach, Three-cornered Jack, Cat Head

Emex australis

DISTRIBUTION Native of South Africa and now widespread. Naturalized throughout Australia. Declared noxious in Australia, USA, Japan and New Zealand.

HABITAT Serious weed of crops and pastures also found in sporting fields, parklands and gardens.

DESCRIPTION

Annual, hairless herb with long, fleshy taproot. Adult plant prostrate with ribbed stems that radiate from crown in all directions.

LEAVES First leaves oval and subsequent leaves are more triangular.

FLOWERS Inconspicuous in clusters in leaf axil. Flowers spring and early summer.

FRUIT/SEED Seedpods grow in clusters with each of the three outer segments forming a spike. Seeds green turning brown as dries.

USES

EDIBLE/OTHER Introduced as a pot herb from South Africa to Western Australia. Travelled across Australia in record time! Worth rediscovering as a spinach substitute tasting similar. Young plants produce large crops of tender leaves, ideal for greens in recipes. I use them until they flower then pull them out before the burrs come. I've had too many punctured bare feet.

MEDICINAL In Africa, Zulus use this herb for stomach disorders and colic and the Xhosa tribe use the herb to relieve digestive troubles and to stimulate appetite.

FARM/ENVIR. Reduces crop yields substantially and contaminates produce. Serious weed of South Africa and Australia, millions of hectares infested. It is a weak competitor and out competed by grasses and legumes. However, will dominate in times of drought or

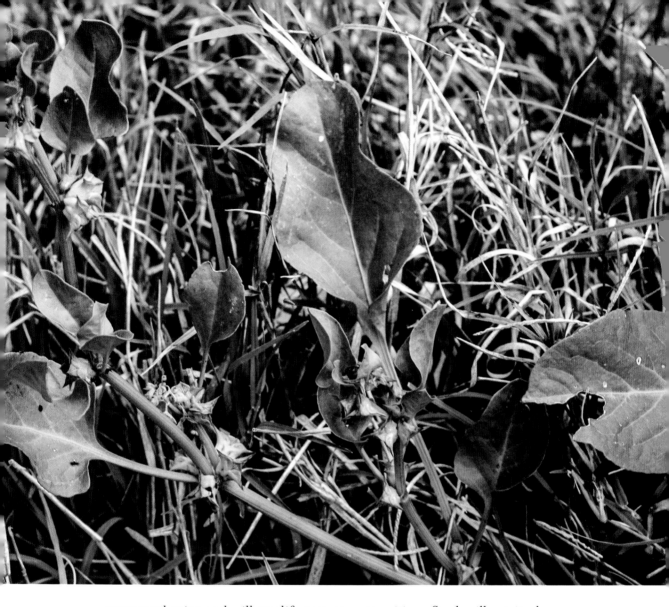

unseasonal rains and will modify pasture composition. Stock will eat it when young. Tough spines cause lameness in stock especially ewes and lambs and even dogs have to wear leather boots when working with the stock. It is a food source in South Africa for the ostrich and in Western Australia the inland Red-tailed Cockatoo and to a lesser extent the Major Mitchell cockatoo, galahs and corellas. Does threaten some flora habitats in National Parks.[174] In South Africa herb used for threadworm in horses.

MAY BE CONFUSED WITH Devil's Thorn (*E. spinosa*) which has fruits half the size and spines half as long and not as widespread as *E. australis*.

FURTHER READING Cytotoxic and antimicrobial activities of *Emex spinosa* (L.) Campd. extract.[175]

WARNING Contains oxalic acid eat in moderation.

STAGGER WEED

Corn Woundwort, Field Woundwort, Field Hedge Nettle

Stachys arvensis

DISTRIBUTION Native of Europe, North Africa and western Asia, now grows worldwide. Naturalized throughout Australia.

HABITAT Grows in low-lying places such as depressions, ditches, creek-sides, borders of swamps and cultivation.

DESCRIPTION

Weak, spreading, hairy annual with four-sided stems and a specific scent.

LEAVES Oval, light green and opposite with wrinkled margins.

FLOWERS Pale pink, grouped in circles round the upper part of the stem. One circle above each pair of leaves.

FRUIT/SEED Small and numerous.

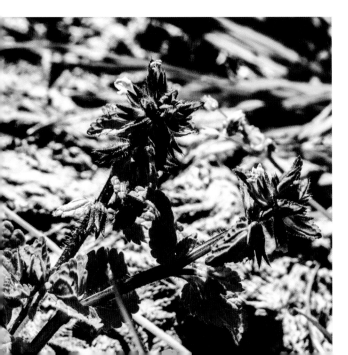
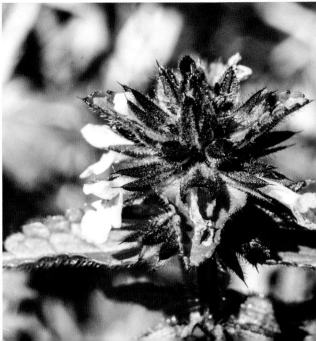

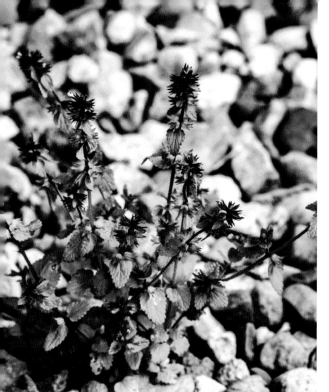
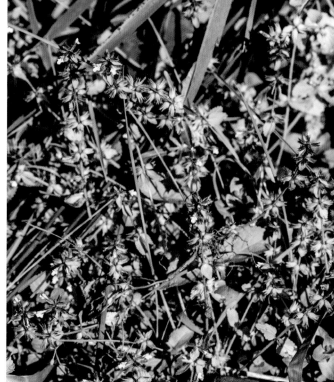

USES

EDIBLE/OTHER Not eaten (unknown toxin).

MEDICINAL Closely related to Wood Betony (*Stachys officinalis*) which was held in high repute in the Middle Ages and by Greeks who extolled its virtues. Sovereign remedy for maladies of the head especially for all types of headaches, calmed the nerves and as a tonic. Has many other uses.[176] Does have side effects such as digestive problems.[177]

FARM/ENVIR. This is an environmental weed in New South Wales, Victoria and Western Australia and a weed of crops. Serious weed in some other countries. It is intolerant of dense shade and likes acidic soils. If you wish to deter the growth of this plant get rid of any damp areas that it likes to grow in and introduce stronger crops/pastures. This plant is believed to cause staggers in cattle, horse and sheep. This unknown toxin seems to be seasonal and varies in different countries. Reports of toxicity especially in sheep have come from Australia. Observations by botanist J Maiden of Australia in the late nineteenth century and early twentieth century were that it was 'good food for milking cows, though if eaten by horses and cattle while engaged at work causes trembling and loss of the use of their limbs'.[178] Goats are used as a weed control.[178a]

FURTHER READING A neurological locomotor disorder in sheep grazing *Stachys arvensis*.[179]

WARNING Contains unknown toxins. Avoid animals grazing on infested paddocks. Humans should only have minimal doses.

STINKING ROGER

Mexican Marigold, Stinkweed

Tagetes minuta

DISTRIBUTION Native of South America and now spread throughout the tropics, subtropics and temperate regions in the world. Naturalized in Australia in New South Wales, Queensland and Victoria.

HABITAT Grown as an ornamental, medicine or perfume plant and accidentally has become a weed. Weed of riverbanks, roadsides, disturbed habitat, wasteland, cultivation and pastures.

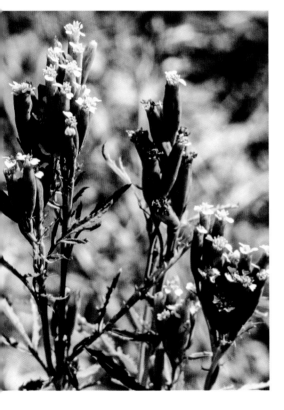

DESCRIPTION

Recognized by its distinct aroma. Tall, woody annual.

LEAVES Deeply divided into narrow, lance-like segments with irregularly-toothed margins. The small brownish oil glands can be seen in the serrations.

FLOWERS Yellow and cylindrical growing in clusters on top of the stems.

SEEDS Narrow black seeds with a tuft of five or six hairs.

USES

EDIBLE/OTHER Grown as a vegetable in Peru and the dried leaves used as a condiment and for flavoring in different food products. Many people find the smell of this plant offensive but I love it, reminding me of fond memories on the farm

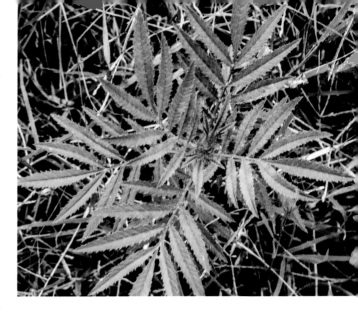

of my childhood. This plant grew in abundance all over the farm and I loved to crush and smell it. The essential oil that is distilled from the leaves is actually highly valued in the perfume trade in France and America. When diluted is a pleasant smell likened to passionfruit or apples. Used commercially to flavor sweets and desserts.

MEDICINAL Used as an insect repellent and control of parasites, especially in Africa where they stuff their mattresses with it. Used for ringworm, parasites and is strongly antifungal. Use as a fresh plant or distilled. Other uses are for fevers, coughs, digestive problems, a mild laxative, rheumatism and for internal and external ulcers. I pick the leaves and tops just as it is flowering and put them into olive oil to make an oil infusion. I do this several times to make it potent then use it in insect repellent sprays and creams. Very good results on mosquitoes. You will also get good results if you crush the plant and rub it directly onto your skin.

FARM/ENVIR. This is a weed of 19 crops in 35 countries as it competes with crops and interferes with their management or harvest. Significant crop seed contaminant especially in East Africa. Environmental weed in Australia. Each plant may have 29,000 seeds/plant and has rapid growth. Livestock will eat it. May taint cow's milk. Cultivated for essential oil and intercropped in corn, tomato and geranium crops. Root secretions have an insecticidal, nematicidal, bacterial and fungicidal effect. Research on intercropping continues. Has agricultural potential. Deters blowfly, mosquitoes, red ant and chicken mite. Use the dried herb ground as a powder or apply as a spray. Hang plants indoors to drive away cockroaches.

MAY BE CONFUSED WITH Cobblers Pegs (*Bidens pilosa*) and Spanish Needles (*Bidens bipinnata*). Stinking Roger is taller, less branched and stronger smelling.

FURTHER READING Antimicrobial activity of flavonoids from leaves of *Tagetes minuta*.[180] The effect of fractionated *Tagetes* oil volatiles on aphid reproduction.[181] Isolation of the insecticidal components of *Tagetes minuta* (Compositae) against mosquito larvae and adults.[182]

WARNING Toxicology of pure compounds isolated from *Tagetes minuta* essential oils. Essential oil must be limited to 0.01% (International Fragrance Association). Skin irritation to agricultural workers working with infested crops.

ST. JOHN'S WORT

St. John's Blood, Witch's Berb

Hypericum perforatum

DISTRIBUTION Native to Europe and western Asia and now worldwide in temperate zones.

HABITAT Grows in open land in semi-dry soils of various sorts but particularly calcareous soils.

DESCRIPTION

An erect perennial up to 1 m (3 ft 3 in) high with a woody, creeping root. Spreads from runners. Has reddish branches.

LEAVES Lance-like, opposite, greener on topside of leaf than underneath, growing directly on the branches and sprinkled with oil glands. Held to the light they look like perforations.

FLOWERS Bright yellow with five petals dotted with small, black oil glands held in three bundles at the end of the stems. Flowers in summer.

FRUIT/SEED Sticky, three-celled capsule with numerous seeds.

USES

EDIBLE/OTHER Used for medicinal purposes. Makes a soothing cup of tea.

MEDICINAL A valuable medicinal herb, one of my favorites. I pick the tops and flowers in late spring and create infused oils, ointments, creams, tinctures, dried herb for tea

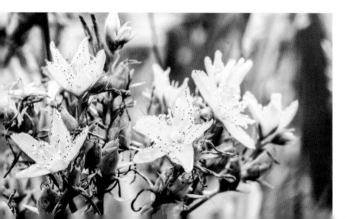
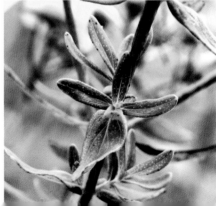

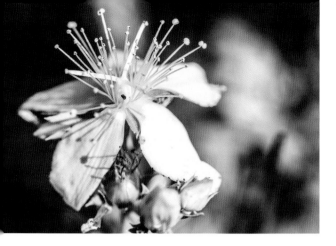
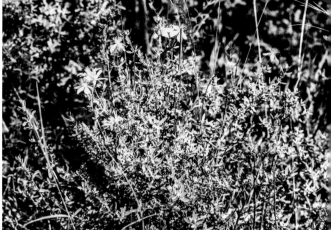

and capsules. This herb is widely researched and has numerous evidence-based uses: an antidepressant including obsessive compulsive disorder and menopause; nerve problems including nerve pain such as neuralgia and headaches; anti-inflammatory internal and external; anticonvulsant; antifungal, antibacterial, antiviral including herpes; digestive system and hormonal herb especially for PMT and excellent protection for the nervous system. Externally I get wonderful results for tension headaches, stings, bites, rashes, skin problems and wherever the nerve endings are damaged including allergic skin reactions. Had good results with phantom pains, injuries, puncture wounds, burns and general muscle aches.[183] It is a noxious weed in New South Wales but I go to properties that only use biological control methods.

FARM/ENVIR. This weed has established itself particularly on dry soils with a shallow layer of topsoil and poor humus matter. A problematic weed that covers large sections of farms. Stock with white faces, especially sheep and Hereford cattle develop sores all over a swollen face and general skin irritation, even possible death. Horses can become unmanageable. Control by improving soil and dense cropping of subterranean clover. One property where we picked the herb did not overgraze and used goats to manage the scattered plants. In a couple of years, the plant had almost disappeared. The leaf paste is applied to treat septic wounds on stock. This weed has economic potential if grown commercially as a medicinal herb. Indicates soil very low in calcium and phosphate and very high in potassium and magnesium. Low humus and moisture, salty, good drainage and high aluminum.[8]

MAY BE CONFUSED WITH Two garden escapees *H. androsaemum* with broader oval leaves and *H. x moserianum* with larger, narrow, oval leaves. Two native species *H. gramineum* and *H. japonicum* with finer leaves.

FURTHER READING See evidence-based references.[183]

WARNING Causes photosensitization in animals and humans. In humans, interaction with other medications. Problem is dose dependent if contains less than 50–10 mg hypericin few side effects will occur. Keep doses at dried herb 2–5 g/day and liquid extract 1:2 3–6 ml/day.

STORKSBILL

Common and Musky Storksbill or Filaree

Erodium cicutarium and *Erodium moschatum*

DISTRIBUTION Originates from southern Europe, North Africa and western Asia and now growing worldwide. Naturalized throughout Australia.

HABITAT Widespread growing in gardens, paddocks, pastures, crops and wasteland.

DESCRIPTION

Low-growing, common, winter annual, occasionally biennial. Starts as a rosette then grows more erect as it matures. Hairy stems and leaves.

LEAVES Divided into separate leaflets, deeply toothed, usually halfway to mid vein. Both leaves similar but Common Storksbill leaflets are more deeply lobed, more noticeable in stem leaves.

FLOWERS Five free petals that vary from pink to mauve. They cluster at the top of the flowering stalks and resemble ornamental geranium flowers. Flowers spring and summer.

FRUIT/SEED Immature fruit resembles a stork's head and beak. As it dries it separates into five parts, each having a tail that coils like a corkscrew. Seed is lance-like and hairy and the coiled end drills seed into the soil.

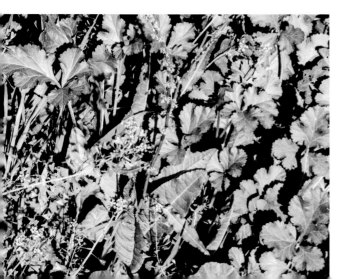
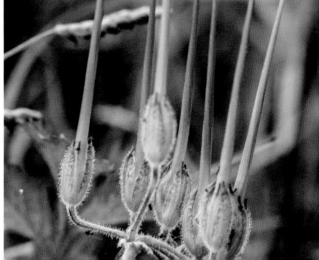

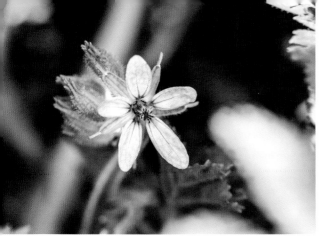
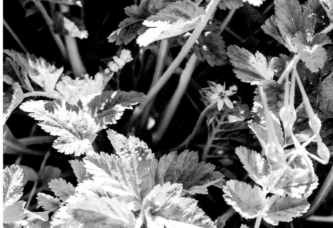

USES

EDIBLE/OTHER Tasty green if picked when young — eat raw or cooked. Common Storksbill is quite palatable but Musky Storksbill has a musky, bitter flavor. Good green dye.

MEDICINAL Common Storksbill has been in use for medicinal purposes for centuries. Antioxidant, antiseptic, antiviral, has astringent properties and a good tonic. Root infusion for stomachache. Use the chewed root for sores and rashes and the whole plant, good for lactation. Leaves also used for typhoid fever.[184] Other countries use it as a kidney tonic, diuretic and anti-inflammatory. Musky Storksbill's main use is for fevers and dysentery.

FARM/ENVIR. Pioneers of disturbed land. Fierce competitors that crowd out or out compete natives. Numerous seeds germinate during the cooler weather and grow thick rosettes that prevents sunlight reaching other seedlings of a later germination. Interferes with establishment of perennial grasses. Invades conservation areas and threatens crop production with economic losses. Common Storksbill makes excellent forage for all kinds of stock and is a valuable hay plant. Musky Storksbill is also edible but most stock avoid it as not very palatable. The corkscrew seed head causes injury to stock, damages hides and devalues fleeces. We have both plants growing on our property and our cattle will eat them both but browse more lightly on the musky tasting one. To eradicate you need to grow a stronger pasture crop such as subterranean Clover or Lucerne.

MAY BE CONFUSED WITH Blue Crowfoot (*E. crinitum*) which is a native species with blue flowers and a wider, three-lobed serrated leaf. Long Storksbill (*E. botrys*) with its longer seed head and wider, serrated leaf.

FURTHER READING Chemical composition and antimicrobial activity of *Erodium* species.[185] A pharmacological appraisal of the folk medicinal usage of Pelargonium grossularioides and *Erodium cicutarium*.[186]

WARNING Stock injury due to corkscrew seed heads. Musky Storksbill may cause photosensitization in sheep if they eat large amounts.

SWEET BRIAR

Briar Rose, Eglantine, Wild Rose

Rosa rubiginosa/Rosa arabica Crép/Rosa eglanteria L.

DISTRIBUTION Native of Europe and western Asia now spread into temperate and cooler subtropical regions. Naturalized mainly in south-eastern Australia.

HABITAT Introduced as an ornamental that has spread into grasslands, gullies, pastures, roadsides, hills and hedgerows.

DESCRIPTION

Perennial, deciduous shrub up to 3 m (10 ft) high. The prickly stems arch away from the woody crown. Stems and leaves often have a brownish-red tint.

LEAVES Five to seven oval leaflets that have serrated margins. Sticky hairs on the undersides and along the margins. Foliage is fragrant especially after a shower of rain.

FLOWERS Small, rose-shaped, with five petals of pale pink. They form loose clusters at the end of the branch. Flowers in spring and summer with little fragrance.

FRUIT/SEED The hip is egg-shaped of a bright orangey-red. Base of the fruit is adorned with bristles and/or spines. Full of hard seeds with irritating hairs. Matures in autumn and early winter.

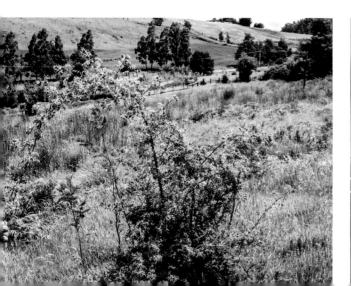
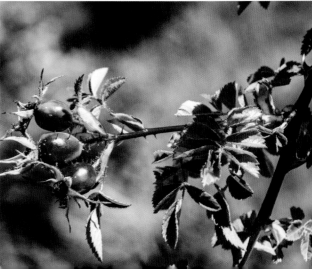

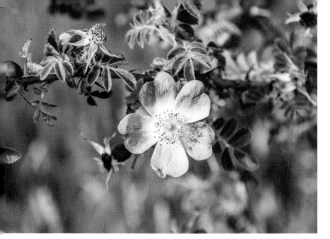
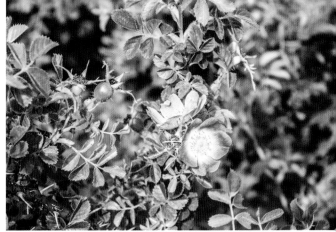

USES

EDIBLE/OTHER Renowned as an excellent source of vitamin C. Yields 450–830 mg vit C/100 g of whole fruit compared to 50 mg/100 g in oranges. The vitamin is partially lost with drying. The hips may be eaten raw but have little flesh; best made into syrups, soups, jellies, jams or tea. Always use a fine sieve to get rid of those irritating hairs. The young shoots are an acceptable vegetable, once candied as a delicacy. The beautiful fragrance is difficult to obtain so an extract perfume of a mixture of floral essences has been created as a copy. The commercial rosehip oil is made from Dog rose (*R. canina*) and is very popular in skin products.

MEDICINAL I make a syrup from the rose hips and mix this with other herbs to make a palatable medicine for children's colds and flu. Also used for gastrointestinal tract problems. Use the roots for colds, cough and flu and the seeds are a good astringent so you can use them for diarrhea, dysentery, hemorrhoids and disorders of the urinary tract. High in antioxidants. Rosehip tea has recently become popular for problems such as arthritis. Commercial rosehips are sourced from other species of roses.

FARM/ENVIR. Significant environmental weed as it invades lowland grassland, forests and alpine regions. In Australia, impacts in Natural Resource Management regions. When I go wildcrafting I have to travel into the hilly areas around our district to find these plants. Goats love eating this plant but other stock usually avoid it. Still popular in cottage gardens, especially in England, and grown as a hedging plant. Small birds find these bushes a safe haven.

MAY BE CONFUSED WITH Rosa species naturalized such as the pink-flowering rambling Dog Rose (*R. canina*) that has hairless flower stalks and fruit and white-flowering, bristly McCartney Rose (*R. bracteata*).

FURTHER READING Carotenoid pigments in *Rosa mosqueta* hips, an alternative carotenoid source for foods.[187] Flavonoid and organic acid content in rose hips (high flavonoids).[188]

WARNING Beware of irritating hairs in the hips.

TANSY

English Fern, Golden Buttons, Scented Fern

Tanacetum vulgare

DISTRIBUTION Native to eastern and central Europe as far as temperate Asia, then spread by man through America, Australia and New Zealand. Naturalized in eastern and southern Australia.

HABITAT Grown for medicinal and ornamental purposes. It has escaped cultivation and now grows wild in natural and secondary vegetation.

DESCRIPTION

Aromatic, perennial, straggling plant 60–120 cm (2–4 ft) tall. Short, stout rootstock.

LEAVES Alternate, fern-like leaves with saw-toothed margins.

FLOWERS Flat top, clusters of golden yellow discs growing on the top of the plant. Strongly scented. Starts flowering in late summer of the second year.

FRUIT/SEED Small seeds, one plant may produce 12,500 seeds but they need open soil to germinate.

USES

EDIBLE/OTHER Used as a flavoring agent in food and beverages and the tea has a calming effect. Oil or powdered Tansy used as an insecticide and in the past, meat was covered in the powder as a deterrent and it was even put in coffins for the same purpose. Cut flowers popular with florists, the essential oil used in perfumery and leaf tips used for cosmetics and ointments.

MEDICINAL Main use is for worming but only use for short durations.[189] I have used this in small doses, it is intensely bitter, but it did work well. Traditionally it was used for a wide variety of problems such as for digestion, nerves, rheumatism and TB [190] but the oil in Tansy is toxic so it must be treated with caution. In research, the essential oil is

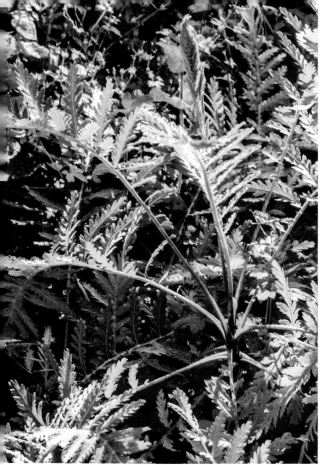
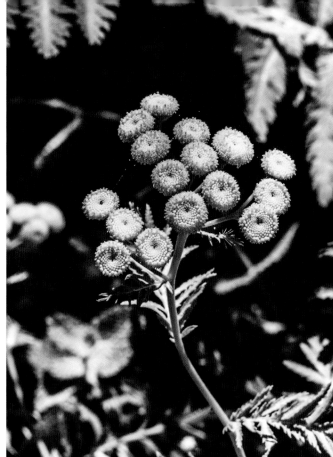

being tested and found to be an effective insecticide. Also showing good results against the herpes virus, cancer research and as an antioxidant. It will bring on menses but beware as an abortifacient. Used externally as an antiseptic and anti-inflammatory, being a good wound healer.

FARM/ENVIR. Aromatic and distasteful to animals and not generally considered toxic. However, some animals will graze on it and this will keep it in control. It is also sensitive to cutting and root extraction. Only a minor weed in Australia unlike North America and Canada where it is a noxious weed. I planted this in my garden 30 years ago as an insecticidal plant. It was not long before it moved from the garden bed and found a niche near the overflow of the tank. Good companion plant for fruit trees to repel flies and ants. Flowers are an important nectar source for pollinating insects. Indicates soil very low in calcium and phosphate, high in other minerals especially copper. Low humus, poor bacteria and moist soil.[8]

FURTHER READING Tick repellent substances in the essential oil of *Tanacetum vulgare*.[191]

WARNING Small doses only as larger doses an irritant. Abortifacient so avoid if pregnant. Toxicity to animals minimal.

THICKHEAD

Redflower Ragleaf

Crassocephalum crepidioide

DISTRIBUTION Native to tropical Africa now widespread in tropical and subtropical areas. Found in north-east Australia and coastal districts.

HABITAT Found in crops, fallows, orchards, forestry, forest gaps, margins, coastal environs, river banks and open woodlands.

DESCRIPTION

Erect, annual, branched herb, slightly succulent and sparsely hairy up to 1 m (3 ft 3 in) high.

LEAVES Soft, alternate, elliptical, sharply toothed.

FLOWERS Open clusters of cylindrical heads that droop on slender stems. Heads are pinkish to reddish brown tipped. Flowers spring to autumn.

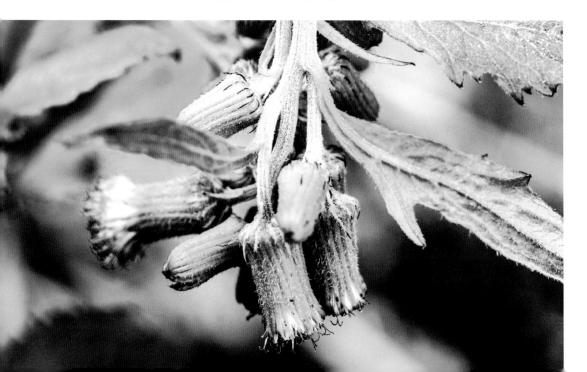

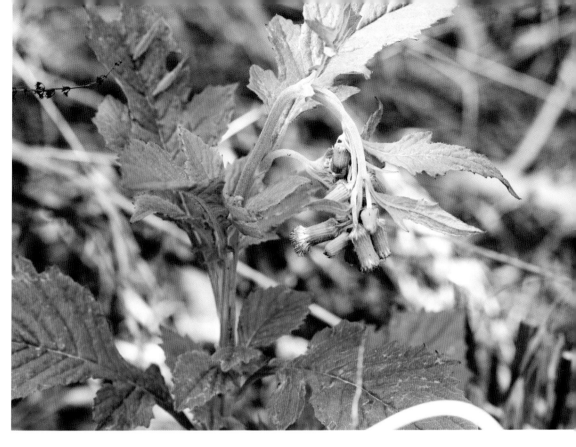

FRUIT/SEED Small gossamer balls contain seeds that fly away on 'parachutes'.

USES

EDIBLE/OTHER Leaves and stems are tender, succulent and mucilaginous. Use as a fresh or cooked vegetable. One of the nicer tasting greens, I quite like the slightly slimy consistency of the leaves, which is not noticeable when eaten with other vegetables.

MEDICINAL Headache, digestive problems and use the juice for constipation. Externally use a poultice of the leaves or make into an ointment or cream for sores, cuts, wounds and injuries. Use the roots for swollen lips.

FARM/ENVIR. Classed as one of the most aggressive weeds in tropical and subtropical regions. May form dense thickets displacing native vegetation. A problem in crops in Asia. Good fodder plant for poultry and livestock.

MAY BE CONFUSED WITH Tropical Burnweed (*C. erechtites valerianifolia*) which is a taller plant with deeply divided leaves and flowers yellow-reddish violet. Also an edible plant. Emilia (*Sonchifolia* var. *javanica*) with bright pink flowers that don't droop and hairy leaves.

FURTHER READING Free radical scavenging and hepatoprotective actions of the medicinal herb.[192]

THORNAPPLE

Castor Oil Plant, Devil's Apple, Jimson Weed

Datura stramonium

DISTRIBUTION Native of America and spread throughout warm-temperate and subtropical regions. Naturalized throughout Australia.

HABITAT Growing in open situations on fertile soils, found in pastures, crops, river flats and abandoned cattle yards.

DESCRIPTION

Robust annual up to 2 m (6 ft 6 in) high, many branched, succulent, sticky and strongly aromatic. Fibrous roots.

LEAVES On long stalks, alternate, oval to oblong in outline with an irregular wavy margin.

FLOWERS Trumpet-like, large, white, borne singly in the forks of branches.

FRUIT/SEED Rigid, spiny capsule covered in numerous (100–200) spines with four chambers full of kidney-shaped seeds.

USES

EDIBLE/OTHER Whole plant toxic so do not eat. Ladies used the seeds in the olden days to dilate their pupils. They felt this made them more desirable. I remember my father got a seed in his eye once and it completely dilated it but no after effects. The seed contains the most toxins so thieves and assassins in India used it to produce insensibility in their victims.

MEDICINAL This herb was once used in powders and cigarettes to relieve spasmodic asthma before modern asthma medications become popular. The beneficial effect is due to the presence of atropine, which paralyses the endings of the pulmonary branches, thus relieving spasms. This is for emergencies only as the herb is narcotic and needs to be treated with care. The British Pharmacopoeia of 1983 states that you use leaves and

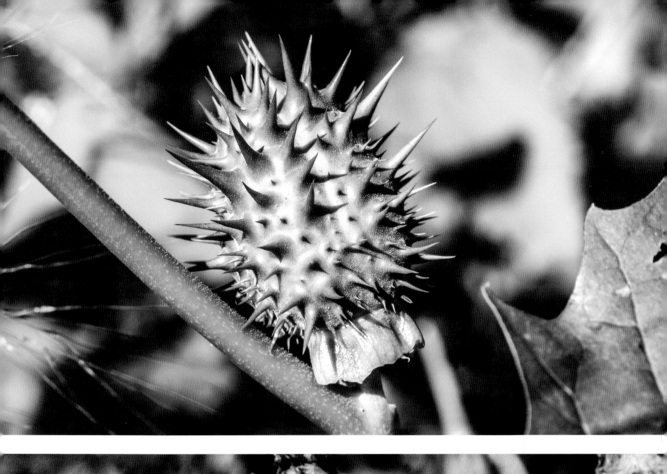
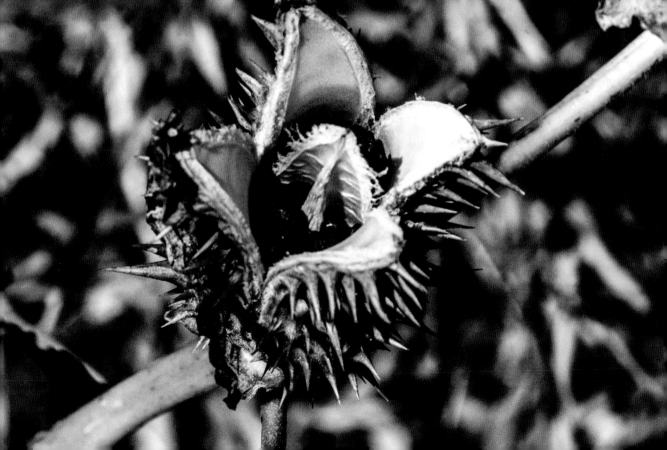

flowering tops only. I use this herb in my Wild Weed ointment and cream due to its ability to relieve spasms and pain. In Ayurvedic, Unani and Sidha medicine they use it to relieve muscular spasm and as a sedative. Flower juice for headaches and leaves are smoked for asthma, cough and as an antimicrobial. Leaf is good for skin diseases, boils, wounds and sores. Crushed leaves will kill bed bugs and crushed seeds in mustard oil for rheumatism. Seeds fried and smoke inhaled through the mouth relieves toothache. Fruit juice applied to scalp for dandruff and falling hair.[193] Alkaloids are extracted for pharmacological use for humans and vet medicine.[194]

FARM/ENVIR. Commonly called by Farmers' Castor oil, which may cause confusion as the true Castor oil plant (*Ricinus communis*) is a 3 m (10 ft) perennial shrub with burr-like groups of fruits. This is a poisonous plant and two to eight seeds may be fatal. Thornapple is also toxic but its toxicity varies with soil type and climate. J Maiden observed that animals that ate small doses of the plant over a period seemed to develop immunity from the toxins.[195] Animals will generally avoid it but I remember our cattle coming down from the top paddock and eating all the leaves off this plant and just leaving the stems and prickly capsules with no ill effects. This is an aggressive plant and large numbers of plants can cover farmland and arable crops. Important to pull up, hoe or slash before plants flower and keep under control. Indicates soil very low in calcium and phosphate and very high in potassium, magnesium and iron. Low in humus, poor in bacteria and drainage plus a soil with a surface crust.[8]

MAY BE CONFUSED WITH Fierce Thornapple (*D. ferox*) that has capsules with only 40 to 60 stout spines of unequal size. Also widespread in Australia.

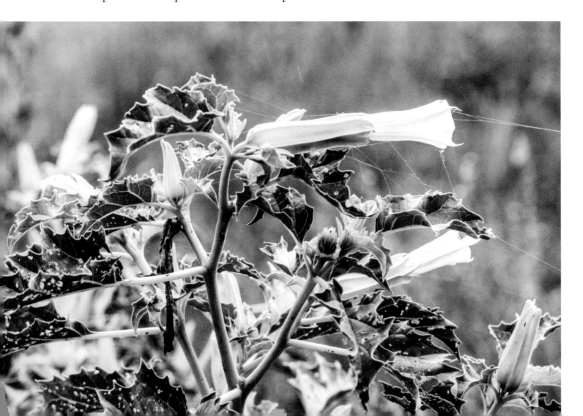

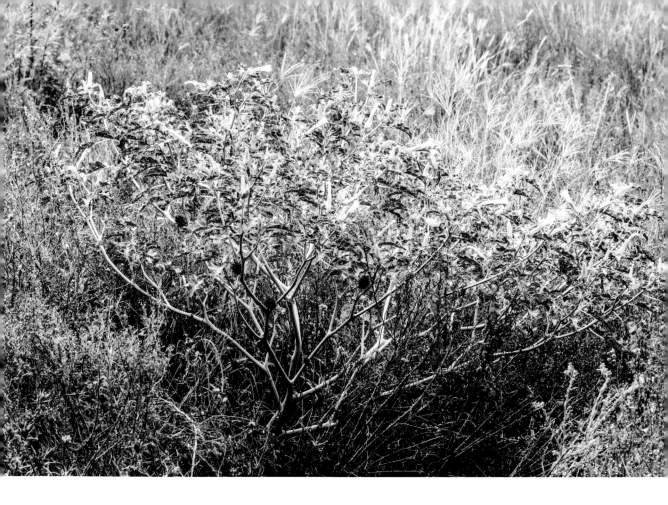

FURTHER READING Phytochemical screening and antimicrobial assessment of *Abutilon mauritianum*, *Bacopa monnifera* and *Datura stramonium*.[196] Pharmacological properties of *Datura stramonium* L. as a potential medicinal tree.[197]

WARNING All the plant is toxic. Use small doses as medicine only. Potentially fatal to stock but most stock avoid it or have built up an immunity.

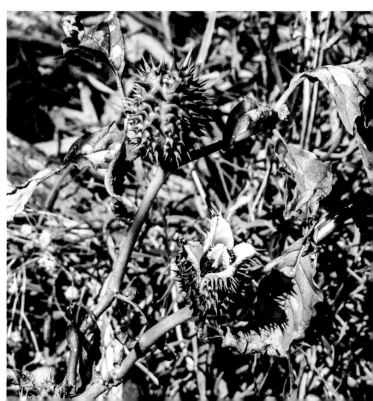

VARIEGATED THISTLE

St Mary's Thistle, Milk Thistle

Silybum marianum

DISTRIBUTION Originated in North Africa, southern Europe and western Asia, now naturalized in temperate regions throughout the world and Australia.

HABITAT Mainly a weed of fertile soils often localized around stock camps and yards. Weed of cultivation or pasture.

DESCRIPTION

Annual or biennial tall plant that starts with a rosette of leaves before producing a strong-branched stem with clasping leaves.

LEAVES Dark green, spiny leaves that are large and broad with pronounced milky variegation, shiny above and duller below.

FLOWERS Large, purple heads up to 13 cm (5 in) across including sharp spines. Solitary at end of branches flowering spring/summer.

FRUIT/SEED Black or brown and are carried away in the wind with their parachutes.

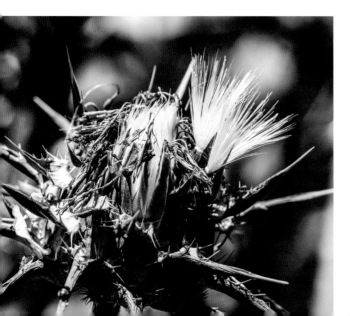
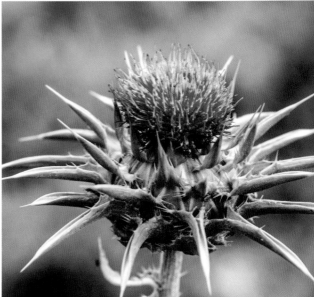

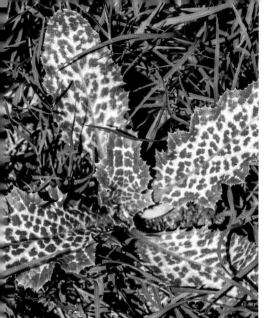
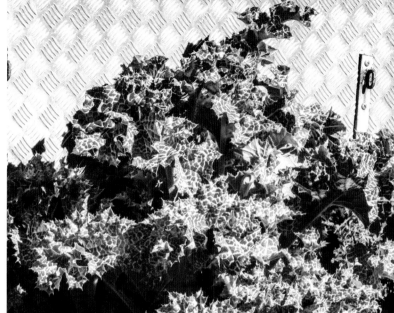

USES

EDIBLE/OTHER Eat young shoots in spring before leaves get prickly, use roots like parsnips, heads like artichokes (rather small and very spiky) and young leaves as well. I think they have the tastiest stems, rather like asparagus. May be eaten raw or cooked once you have cleaned off the clasping leaves.

MEDICINAL Renowned liver tonic, first used by Dioscorides in AD 50. This protective and safe herb treats hepatitis, fatty liver, liver damage, allergies and digestive, cholesterol and skin problems. Protects the liver from chemotherapy and externally from sun damage. Seeds contain medicinal qualities. Collect just before seeds are ready to disperse and birds appear. The spikes can be lethal so be careful. I cut off the heads and my husband pulls them apart with pliers. Dry, grind and eat (in general a teaspoon a day), put into capsules, make tincture, decoctions or creams.

FARM/ENVIR. It loves rich, black, fertile soils high in nitrogen, particularly on dairy farms. Before slashers became available infested farms would sell at reduced prices. Now farmers keep the number of thistles to a minimum using strong crops like Lucerne to compete. However, like all weeds they may be a friend or a foe. One wheat farmer I know had an infestation of this herb and made a profit from it. Using his wheat harvester, he made more money from exporting the seed for medicinal purposes than he got for his wheat. Safely eaten by stock except when slashed and wilted, at this time keep stock out of this area.

FURTHER READING Adjunct to cancer therapy as it cleanses and detoxifies after chemotherapy.[198] Renal protective, inflammatory hepatic cirrhosis.[199]

WARNING Nitrate content higher in wilted plants and can cause livestock death.

VERVAIN

Common Verbena

Verbena officinalis

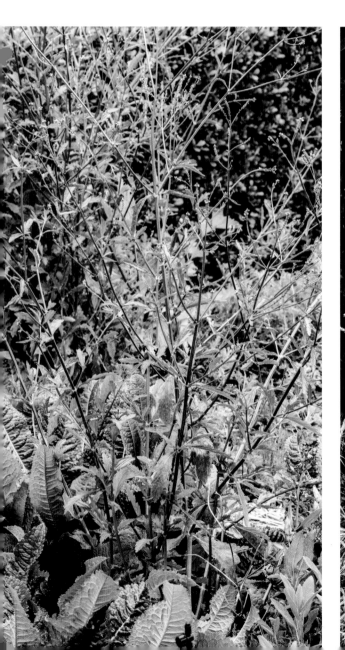
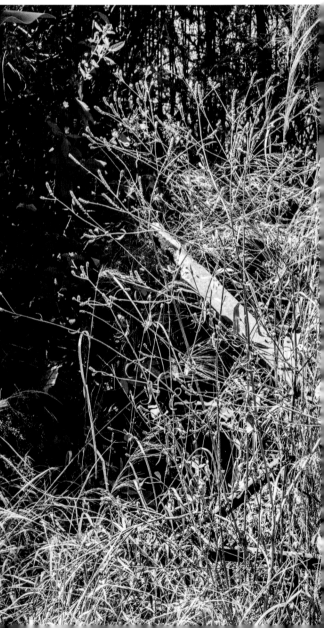

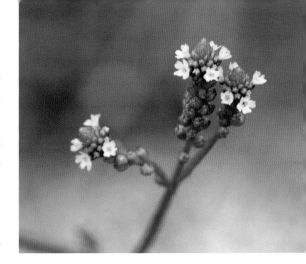

DISTRIBUTION Cosmopolitan and naturalized throughout Australia, especially the eastern region.

HABITAT Roadsides, arable land, disturbed areas in rainforests, disturbed ground and in sunny pastures. It avoids shady areas.

DESCRIPTION

Weedy, perennial 35–80 cm high with angular stems.

LEAVES Widely spaced and unevenly dissected leaves in opposite pairs.

FLOWERS Slender, sparsely flowered spikes of small, lilac flowers. Self-fertile, flowering in the warmer months. Harvest when flowering and dry immediately.

FRUIT/SEEDS Tiny seeds.

USES

EDIBLE/OTHER Revered by the druids and known as a magic herb during the Middle Ages. Legend says this herb was used to staunch the wounds of Jesus. Parboil, season and eat these rough leaves and use the flowers as a garnish. I prefer to use the leaves in a relaxing tea. Taste is slightly bitter and astringent.

MEDICINAL Used medicinally for hundreds of years. Mainly used as a sedative, for nervous disorders, anxiety and insomnia. Helps make mother's milk and used for kidney and bladder complaints. Externally, treats minor injuries and sores. In China, used for its antibacterial, anti-inflammatory, antidepressant and antitumor activity. Used as a capsule, tea, tincture or extract. The tea I have used has a mild effect, the extract is more potent.

FARM/ENVIR. Grown in gardens where it attracts bees and butterflies. I started this herb in my garden but like a lot of garden escapee weeds it now grows in a few clumps in the paddock. It doesn't normally form dense stands; a minor weed. Indicates soil very low in calcium, phosphate and high in potassium.[8]

MAY BE CONFUSED WITH Inland Verbena (*V. africana*) whose lower leaves are toothed and never dissected. Native Verbena (*V. gaudichaudii*) – flower head is distinctly glandular.

FURTHER READING Studied for their effects on experimental risk factors for urinary stones.[200] Anti-inflammatory and analgesic activity of the topical preparation.[201]

VIOLET, SWEET

Sweet-scented, Common and English violet

Viola odorata

DISTRIBUTION Native to Asia, North Africa and Europe. Now widespread and naturalized in southern Australia.

HABITAT Garden escapee loving damp, fertile soils in a shady position. Found in gardens, adjoining lands, woodlands and wastelands.

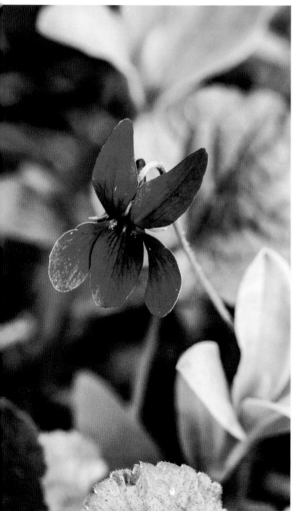

DESCRIPTION

Perennial 10–15 cm (4–6 in) tall on short rhizomes. Stemless.

LEAVES On end of stems that arise from creeping rhizomes. Heart shaped leaves.

FLOWERS Stalks arise from forks of the leaf stems and bear single, deep purple flowers, some variations occur. All are scented. Mostly flowers in spring.

FRUIT/SEED Light brown, oval seeds.

USES

EDIBLE/OTHER Edible flowers and leaves. Eat raw or cook the leaves, it will thicken soups. Flowers may be used as a coloring agent for drinks and syrups. They impart odor and color in vinegars. In addition, you can crystallize the flowers to decorate cakes. I like eating the flowers fresh and using them to decorate my salad or fruit dishes.

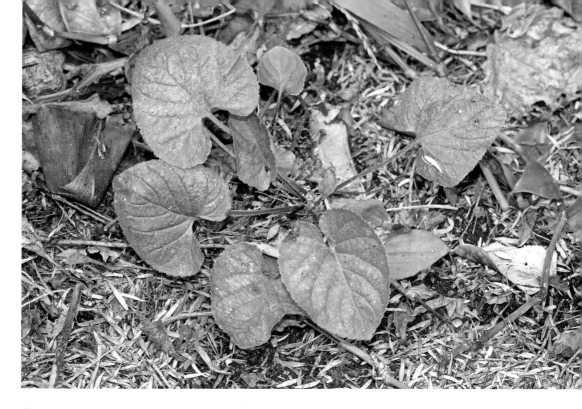

Grown in southern France for the perfume industry. Once violet water and perfumes were the most popular scents in England.

MEDICINAL Main use is in the treatment of respiratory disorders especially bronchitis, asthma, chronic nasal problems and catarrh. Use in cough mixtures, for sore throats, headaches, fever and bleeding piles. Externally used for skin diseases. I use the leaves in my protective lip salve as it protects lips from wind chaffs, the occurrence of lip cancers, cracked and sore lips. One woman with a long-term sore on her lip applied the fresh crushed leaf regularly and it healed within a few weeks.

FARM/ENVIR. Common environmental weed in Victoria and South Australia and a minor weed in New South Wales and Western Australia. They grow in large clumps, which are easy to pull up to keep this plant under control. I have a large area under some bushes at work where they have spread and do well as long as I keep them moist. Indicates soil low in calcium and manganese.[8]

MAY BE CONFUSED WITH Native Violets (*V. hederacea*) with their smaller leaves and white and purple flowers — edible flowers. Many Viola cultivars of various colors have been bred, none are medicinal.

FURTHER READING Antipyretic studies on some indigenous Pakistani medicinal plants.[202] The effectiveness of *Viola odorata* in the prevention and treatment of formalin-induced lung damage in the rat.[203] Anticancer and chemosensitizing abilities of cycloviolacin O2 from *Viola odorata* and psyle cyclotides from *Psychotria leptothyrsa*. Biopolymers.[204]

WANDERING JEW

Common Wandering Jew and Scurvy Weed

Tradescantia fluminensis (albiflora), Commelina cyanea

DISTRIBUTION Both plants often called Wandering Jew. The Common Wandering Jew is native to South America and now grows worldwide. Naturalized in south-eastern Australia. Scurvy weed is a native and widespread in New South Wales and Queensland.

HABITAT Both are garden weeds from the Commelinaceae family, which inhabit shady areas, older and neglected gardens, bushland, forest margins, wasteland, roadside and ditches.

DESCRIPTION

Both plants are trailing, perennial, succulent herbs that grow from the nodes. Both frost tender.

LEAVES Dark green, alternate, broadly lance-like, smooth and semi-glossy growing directly from the stems.

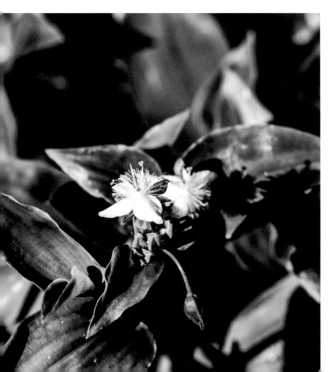
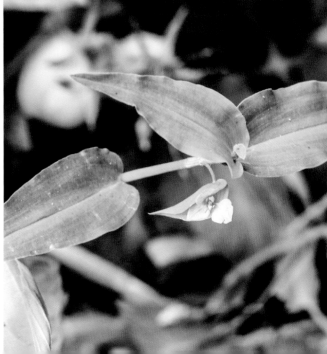

FLOWERS Enclosed pod on a stalk opens to reveal three white, oval-shaped petals in Common Wandering Jew and three blue, oval-shaped flowers in Scurvy Weed.

FRUIT/SEED Common Wandering Jew does not seed. Scurvy Weed is a capsule with two to five seeds.

USES

EDIBLE/OTHER The crunchy, pleasant tasting leaves from both plants are edible and I enjoy eating them in salads or cooked. Early white settlers ate Scurvy Weeds and, as the name suggests, they believed the plant possessed a good source of vitamin C. The vitamin content of this plant has not been assessed. Common Wandering Jew is eaten more rarely but there are many accounts of its usage.

MEDICINAL Closely related is *C. communis*, which is used for epidemic flu and upper respiratory tract infections, acute tonsillitis, pharyngitis, dysentery, edema, difficult urination and conjunctivitis. Use as a tea or juice. Externally the crushed plant is applied topically for boils, carbuncles, insect bites and burns. Chewed into a small wad and packed over mouth ulcers gives relief.

FARM/ENVIR. Common Wandering Jew is a significant environmental weed in Australia and a priority in four Natural Resource Management regions. Stock eat these plants and it is a favorite with my chooks. I grow it under my fruit trees to help retain moisture. These plants are over 90% water and readily obtain moisture from any dew or moisture in the area. When the tree's moisture level drops this ground cover will keep the roots moist. Important in dry climates, especially in droughts when the water supply is unreliable. It cuts down my watering by at least 30%. It will form thick mats that smother other plantings depriving them of light. My garden is covered in this plant so I am constantly pulling it up to stop it competing with my existing plants. Easy to pull up but hard to eradicate as if you leave a small piece of root it will regrow.

MAY BE CONFUSED WITH Other plants in this species are Asiatic dayflower (*C. communis*) with two upper blue petals and a smaller, white lower petal. This plant grows in Eurasia and North America, rarer in Australia and has medicinal uses. Hairy Wandering Jew (*C. benghalensis*) a more hairy plant that is eaten in Asia. Growing on north coast of Australia. Other *Commelina* natives such as *C. ensifolia*, *C. lanceolata* and *C. undulatus* are also edible.

FURTHER READING Effect of aqueous and methanol extracts of *Tradescantia zebrine* and *fluminensis* on human cells.[205]

WARNING Some sensitive dogs have a skin allergy to these plants.

WATERCRESS

Common or English Watercress

Rorippa nasturtiumaquaticum/Nasturtium officinale

DISTRIBUTION Native to Europe and now widespread. Now naturalized in southern and eastern Australia.

HABITAT Found in shallow, muddy water, swamps, drains, soaks, slow-running creeks and small streams.

DESCRIPTION

Semi-aquatic, hairless perennial with angular, hollow stems. Roots at the nodes. Often seen floating and forming large clumps of matted roots underwater.

LEAVES Succulent, round-to-oval leaves made up of three to nine segments, terminal one is the largest.

FLOWERS Small, white with four petals, similar to other Brassica flowers. Flowers summer to mid-autumn.

FRUIT/SEED Sausage-shaped seedpods that are held upright on the stems and each half of the pod has two rows of seeds.

USES

EDIBLE/OTHER Collect from clear, flowing streams that have no stock along their upper reaches. The liver fluke, which is a parasite that comes from stock, lives in polluted water in the hollow stems of watercress. I collect plants and grow them in my water feature at home, so I know they are free from this parasite. Collect the older leaves, which have a stronger, peppery taste than younger leaves. Use them in salads or put them in a dish at the end of cooking. If you are concerned about the parasite then cook this herb as cooking kills it. Makes a delicious summer soup. In the UK this plant is going through

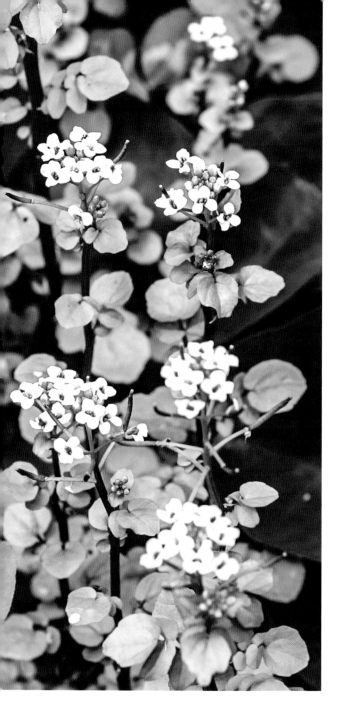

a renaissance where people grow large amounts in fresh flowing water. The herb is collected for markets and customers eat it fresh or juice it.

MEDICINAL For centuries, this plant was an official medicine. Rich in vitamins and minerals especially Vitamins A, B2, C, D and E, beta-carotene, iron, iodine, sulfur, calcium and amino acids. Renowned for its antiscorbutic qualities and as a general tonic. Used for the respiratory system for asthma, TB and makes an excellent cough remedy when mixed with honey. Good for diarrhea and digestive problems and externally for boils, sores, abscesses, mouth ulcers, gingivitis and even baldness. It is antiviral, good against parasites, obesity, fluid retention, anorexia and for liver and gall.

FARM/ENVIR. Cultivated for the markets in many countries although in Australia mainly found in the wild. Rarely found in our small creek as it dries up in summer. Must have constant moisture. Watercress may block up small watercourses if it has excessive growth, otherwise a weed with minimal impact. With its distinctive peppery flavor and health attributes, this plant should be grown and marketed more extensively in Australia.

MAY BE CONFUSED WITH One-row watercress (*R. microphylla*) which is similar except its fruits have a single irregular row of seeds in each half of the pod. Yellow or marsh cress (*R. palustris*) which has yellow flowers and crinkled, lobed leaves. Both widespread in Australia and edible.

FURTHER READING Influence of nitrogen and sulfur on biomass production and carotenoid and glucosinolate concentrations in Watercress (*Nasturtium officinale* R. Br.).[206] Growth inhibitory activities of crude extracts obtained from herbal plants in the Ryukyu Islands on several human colon carcinoma cell lines.[207]

WARNING Beware of liver fluke.

WATER HYACINTH

Eichhornia crassipes

DISTRIBUTION Native of South America and now widespread in tropical and subtropical regions. Naturalized in Australia in the warmer regions, mostly coastal. Frost tender.

HABITAT In waterways of all types. Cultivated due to its beautiful flowers. It was introduced to numerous creeks, rivers and lakes in warmer climates where it has quickly flourished.

DESCRIPTION

Pretty, erect, aquatic plant up to 1 m (3 ft 3 in) high. At the base of the leaf stalk is a large bulbous-looking development, which is composed of numerous air-cells, which act like a float to support the plant in the water. Roots grow about 1 m (3 ft 3 in) long and it can survive in shallow to very deep water. Grows into enormous mats made up of numerous plants.

LEAVES Glossy, circular to kidney-shape.

FLOWERS Group of pretty flowers arises from a stem. Violet with one petal having a violet blotch with a yellow center. Flowers late summer and autumn and in warmer areas all year round.

FRUIT/SEED Numerous seeds quickly germinate and grow when in contact with the water. In ideal conditions one plant can produce 248 offspring in 90 days.

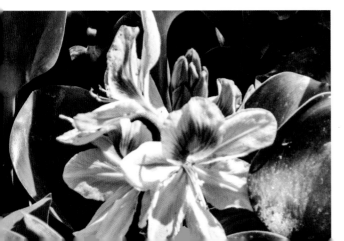
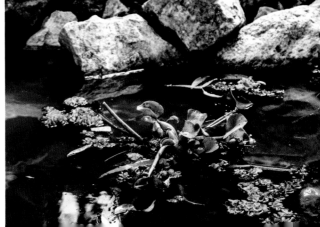

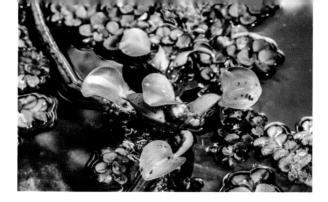
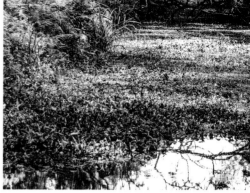

USES

EDIBLE/OTHER The leaves, flower spikes and young bulbous bottoms are edible, boiled or fried. However, try cautiously as fresh plants contain prickly crystals and they can be very irritating. These crystals are in quite a few plants, which I experienced when eating Taro, and I thought I had eaten a mouthful of stinging nettles. Took ages to soothe. Taste is bland although some authors say there is some flavor. You must only collect plants in clean water as the plants accumulate toxins. In Africa the fresh plants are used for cushions in canoes and to plug holes in charcoal bags.

MEDICINAL The juice from the plant is used for treating wounds and this is one of the best plants to help with tumors. Research shows potential for the following – anticancer, antioxidant, antifungal and antibacterial.

FARM/ENVIR. One of the world's worst weeds spread mostly by humans beautifying their waterways. A serious menace to navigation, it blocks waterways, interferes with water flow, fishing and affects paddy crops such as rice. When I went to Vietnam, I could not believe the massive 'islands' of Water Hyacinth in their rivers. Pieces would break off and float down past our boat. When the plant is established the water is rendered unfit for drinking as the decomposing plants give off an offensive smell and water becomes inky black and putrid. Stock will not touch it. When food is scarce, stock will try to eat it but many drownings have occurred in fast moving water. Dense infestations also reduce oxygen levels in the water. The dense monocultures threaten local native-species diversity and change the physical and chemical aquatic environment thus altering the ecosystems. Thus, mechanical methods and herbicides are constantly used to keep it under control. This plant has the ability to absorb chemicals and pollutants including lead, mercury and strontium.[90] Many research papers are showing how useful this plant could be, including using it in wastewater treatment. The plants may be used for composting, fuel bricks, paper, board, animal feed and generating methane biogas.

FURTHER READING Novel rhythms of N_1-acetyl-N_2-formyl-5-methoxykynuramine and its precursor melatonin in Water Hyacinth: importance for phytoremediation.[208] *Eichhornia crassipes* (Mart) solms: From water parasite to potential medicinal remedy.[209] Invasion and control of Water Hyacinth (*Eichhornia crassipes*) in China.[210]

WHITE CEDAR

Chinaberry, Persian or Cape Lilac, Dygal (Aboriginal)

Melia azedarach (M. australasica)

DISTRIBUTION Native to southern Asia and northern Australia and now spread widely due to gardeners growing it for its beauty and hardiness. Widely planted and now naturalized in eastern Australia.

HABITAT Growing in paddocks, wasteland, disturbed sites and roadsides.

DESCRIPTION

Deciduous, medium-sized tree with a rounded canopy. It is fast growing and the trunk is grey-brown with fissures.

LEAVES Lime-green, toothed leaflets.

FLOWERS Bell-shaped, lilac to pink growing in clusters at the end of stems. Honey-scented fragrance. Appear mid-spring.

FRUIT/SEED Dull yellow, round, wrinkled and fleshy. Has black seeds. Stays on the tree all winter.

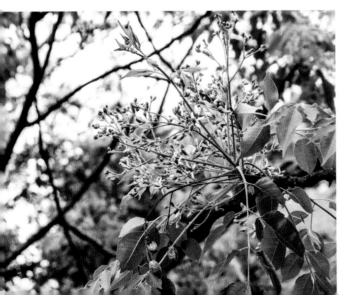
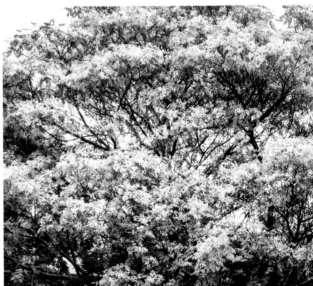

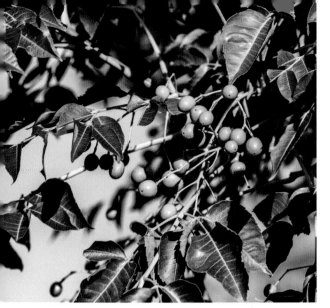
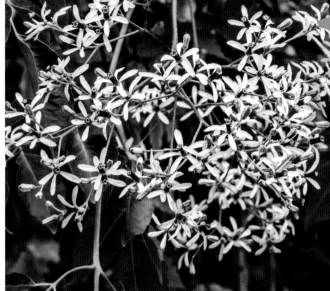

USES

EDIBLE/OTHER Fruits may be toxic and children have died from eating six to eight ripe fruits. However, in some countries people eat the fruits with no side effects.[213] Soft and easily worked timber.

MEDICINAL Used for fevers, parasites, viral infections, scrofula, leprosy, digestive troubles. Also for arthritis, inflammation and autoimmune diseases. Externally psoriasis, eczema, wounds, boils, head lice, pustular eruptions and nervous headaches. Use the oil just like the related Neem oil. Alcoholic and aqueous extracts of flowers and berries are non-toxic to rats and mice up to a dose of 1,500 mg/kg. Intravenous administration led to more severe symptoms at sublethal doses.

FARM/ENVIR. This invading tree needs to be kept under control as birds spread its numerous seeds and it suckers easily. The white cedar moth is its most serious pest as their hairy larvae will quickly strip the leaves off a tree. This tree has established itself in our area. It grows all over farmer's paddocks and beside the road. Often found growing in groups. It is grown as an ornamental tree as it has beautiful flowers with a lovely perfume and makes a good shade tree. Does not seem to cause any problems with stock as they usually avoid eating the seeds.

FURTHER READING Immunomodulatory activities of *Melia azedarach* L. leaf extracts on human monocytes.[211] Antiviral activity of cytotoxicity assays of crude and partly purified extracts of *Melia azedarach* fresh green leaves.[212]

WARNING Fruit may be toxic to humans, the principle is meliatoxin.[213] The fruit is toxic to stock. Pollen may induce allergic respiratory disease. The hairy white cedar moth's larvae will cause irritation if you touch its hairs.

WILD COTTON

Milkweed, Melkbos (S. Africa), Narrow-leaved cotton bush

Gomphocarpus fruticosus/Asclepias fruticosa

DISTRIBUTION Native of South Africa now widespread. Naturalized in southern and eastern Australia.

HABITAT Grown as an ornamental in gardens. Now found in wasteland, pastures, roadsides and wooded areas. Adapts to a wide variety of soils.

DESCRIPTION

Perennial, erect, attractive shrub. Grows to about 1.5 m (5 ft) high with slender stems. Has white, milky latex.

LEAVES Narrow and dull green.

FLOWERS Creamy white, which grow in clusters at the end of stems. Flowering in the warmer months.

FRUIT/SEED Egg-shaped with short, curved beak. Fruits covered in long, soft bristles. When mature the balloons burst open and are full of silky hairs attached to small, black seeds.

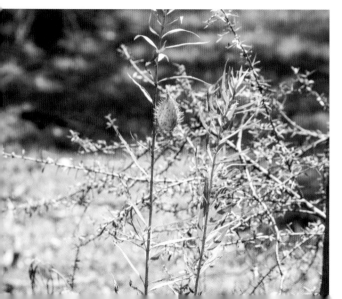
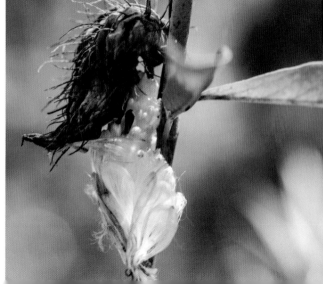

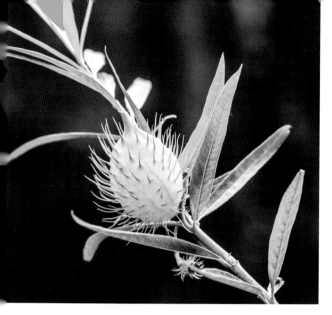 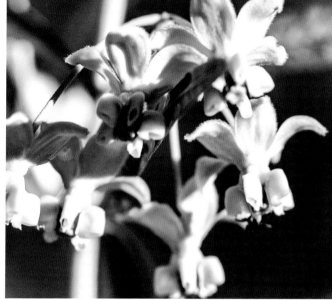

USES

EDIBLE/OTHER The silky hairs are collected to fill pillows. This is a luxury in South Africa and people feel it is worth the effort to fill and create delicate 'melkbos' seed pillows. As a child living on dairy farms this plant was always around and I used to love popping the fruit then collecting the silky down, which is a delight to the skin. Very strong stems which I have used in my Bush Tucker camps as a basis for baskets.

MEDICINAL White milky latex used as an excellent treatment for warts. Zulus make a tea for children's tummy ache and diarrhea and dried leaf as a snuff for TB. Strong brew of leaves is a respected farm remedy for easing distemper in dogs. In the Orange Free State they use the roots for diabetes.[214]

FARM/ENVIR. A serious environmental weed in Australia invading vegetation near waterways and competing with natives. Also invading conservation areas. Dense infestations reduce productivity of pastures. Stock rarely eat this plant but deaths have been recorded in cattle, sheep and poultry due to contaminants in fodder and chaff. Once popular as an ornamental especially the Balloon Cotton Bush. In South Africa, sprays from these plants are sought after by florists. Preferred fruit for the caterpillar of the wanderer butterfly.

MAY BE CONFUSED WITH Balloon Cotton Bush (*G. physocarpus*) which grows in Queensland and north-east New South Wales. Fruits are rounder with a sunken tip and tiny beak. Will hybridize with *G. fruticosus*.

FURTHER READING Ethnopharmacological evaluation of a traditional herbal remedy used to treat gonorrhea.[215] Inhibitory properties of selected South African medicinal plants against Mycobacterium tuberculosis [216]

WARNING Toxic to humans and animals.

WILD RADISH

Jointed Charlock

Raphanus raphanistrum

DISTRIBUTION Native to Europe and now grows worldwide. Naturalized in southern and eastern Australia.

HABITAT Grows on roadsides, pastures and disturbed habitats.

DESCRIPTION

Annual or biennial herb, when young has a rosette of leaves then grows erect with bristly branches. Its fibrous root system grows to a depth of 20 cm (8 in).

LEAVES Alternate, lower leaves covered in rough hairs and deeply divided. Upper leaves smaller.

FLOWERS Terminal with four, pale yellow with purple veins.

FRUIT/SEED Seed pod fleshy, spongy and cylindrical with pointed beak. Contains two to ten oval, orange-brown seeds. Seeds in winter.

USES

EDIBLE/OTHER Related to the domesticated radish this plant has a somewhat hot taste. Eat finely chopped young leaves raw or cooked (older leaves bitter). Eat flower buds like broccoli. Eat seeds raw, cooked, sprouted or ground as mustard substitute. In nineteenth century England Wild Radish was so common the grain was sold as 'Durham mustard', a highly regarded mustard substitute. I find this a lovely green and condiment to enjoy in the winter months. Edible oil from the seeds.

MEDICINAL Seeds for hemorrhoids, malaria and skin disease. In addition, the plant used for rheumatism.

FARM/ENVIR. This plant is the third most widely spread and serious weed of broad acre farming. Often contaminates winter wheat and other crops. Affects winter yields of wheat.

'Bread poisoning' has occurred when wheat was contaminated by large quantities of the seed. In 1997, the weed was in 45 different crops in 65 countries. It is an alternative host for a number of pests and allergens. Ingestion by cattle and sheep may taint the milk.[8] Indicates soil very low in calcium, phosphate and very high in potassium, magnesium and iron. Low in humus, salty, low bacteria, hardpan and contains aluminum.[217]

FURTHER READING Insecticidal activity of four medicinal plant extracts against *Tribolium castaneum*.[218] In vivo anti-inflammatory and in vitro antioxidant activities of Mediterranean dietary plants.[219]

MAY BE CONFUSED WITH Other species of the Brassica family.

WARNING Toxic to stock (especially the seeds) although stock usually avoid eating it.

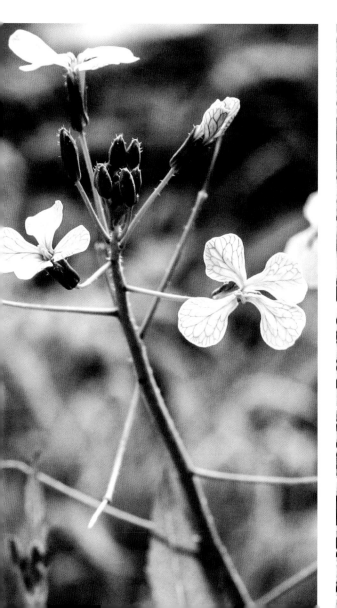
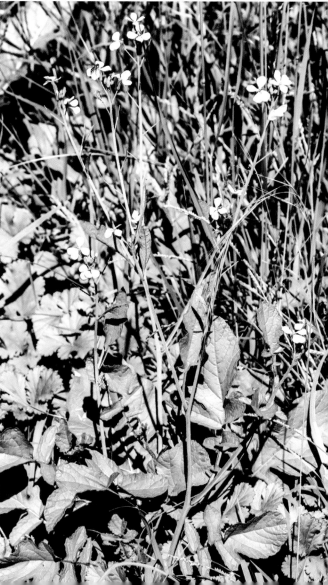

WOOD SORREL

Creeping Oxalis, Yellow Wood Sorrel, Sleeping Clover

Oxalis corniculata

DISTRIBUTION Native to South America and now worldwide. Naturalized throughout Australia.

HABITAT Weed of lawns and pastures and is often found in damp and shady places.

DESCRIPTION

Looking like a miniature clover that has a sharp, sour taste to its leaves. Perennial, prostrate, sprawling, with a creeping rootstock like the mint family.

LEAVES Small, heart-shaped, occur in groups of three. At night, in the rain or if exposed to direct sunlight the leaves fold up.

FLOWERS Bell-shaped, small and yellow with five petals.

FRUIT/SEED Elongated capsules that eject wrinkled seeds some distance when mature.

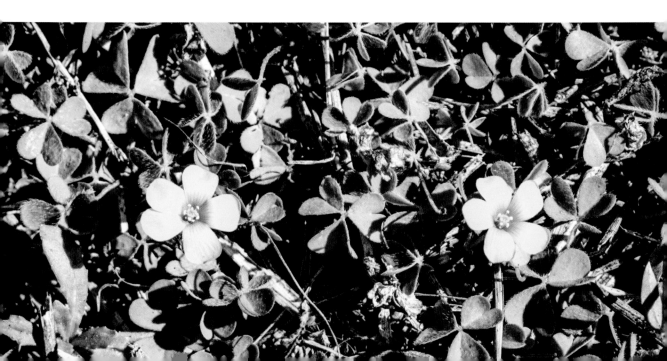

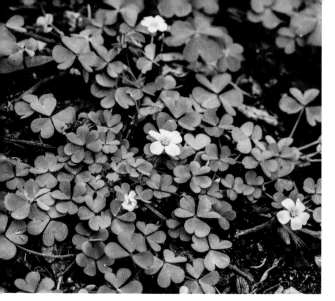
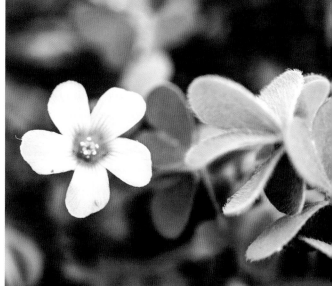

USES

EDIBLE Leaves are a condiment with their sour flavor. I love picking them and using them in salads for a slight zing. If cooking put them in at the end, so you do not lose their delicate flavor. Colonists ate them to stop scurvy and in Tasmania, they were baked into sweet tarts. Once extensively eaten but now replaced by the cultivated sorrel with its large leaves that are so much easier to collect than the fiddly little Wood Sorrel leaves.

MEDICINAL In Ayurvedic, Unani and Sidha medicines they use it externally for burns, muscular and joint pain, to remove warts, rheumatism, cuts, wounds, swellings, insect stings and use the juice for conjunctivitis. Internally for dysentery, diarrhea, jaundice, liver disorders, stomach complaints, convulsions, anorexia, chronic cough, fever and colds.[220] Old herbalists believed that Wood Sorrel was more effective than the true sorrels as a blood cleanser, will strengthen a weak stomach, produce an appetite and check vomiting.

FARM/ENVIR. This plant contains oxalic acid that in large amounts is toxic but the small amounts stock consume does not seem to be a problem. Have a small patch for your private use but keep it under control in your garden, as due to its underground network it can be invasive. However, easy to eradicate with mulch or stronger competition.

MAY BE CONFUSED WITH Sour Sob (*Oxalis pes-caprae*) which has larger, yellow flowers. Pink Shamrock (*Oxalis debilis* Kunth var. *corymbosa*) which has purplish-pink flowers. Both common garden weeds. There are numerous other *Oxalis* species all containing oxalic acid and tasting sour, however, Wood Sorrel is usually much smaller.

FURTHER READING Phytochemical analysis and antibacterial activity of *Oxalis corniculata*.[221] Cardioprotective effects of aqueous extract of *Oxalis corniculata* in experimental myocardial infarction.[222] Pharmacological activity of *Oxalis corniculata*.[223]

WARNING Contains oxalic acid.

YARROW

Staunchweed, Milfoil, Soldiers Woundwort

Achillea millefolium

DISTRIBUTION Native to Europe and Asia and now widespread. Naturalized mainly in south-eastern Australia.

HABITAT Garden escapee growing in wasteland, along roadsides and on unused land.

DESCRIPTION

Aromatic perennial with far-creeping runners forming a dense mat. Erect, furrowed slightly, woolly stems 10–60 cm (4–24 in) high.

LEAVES Slightly hairy leaves divided into fine leaflets. Have a distinct sweet scent similar to chrysanthemums.

FLOWERS Small, white to pink forming dense heads in early summer to autumn.

FRUIT/SEED Dry, single-seeded fruit.

USES

EDIBLE/OTHER Mix with Elder and Peppermint to make a lovely winter tea.

MEDICINAL Renowned for its healing abilities for thousands of years. Its ability to heal wounds and stem the flow of blood was of great importance to armies. This plant has so many constituents it is not surprising it has so many uses. Here are a few uses: anti-inflammatory, antiseptic, respiratory problems, fevers, bedwetting, urinary problems, circulation, digestive problems, cramps, diarrhea, dysentery, hemorrhoids, hayfever, lowers blood pressure, liver, periods, rheumatism, skin wounds and a tonic. I have used the hot Yarrow tea numerous times for cystitis and drunk the tea for colds, flu and fevers with great results.

FARM/ENVIR. Stock will graze on this plant so you will not find it growing in pastures. There is a market for the sale of this plant on a small scale. I have grown large areas of this

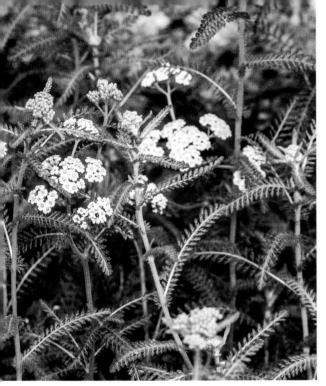
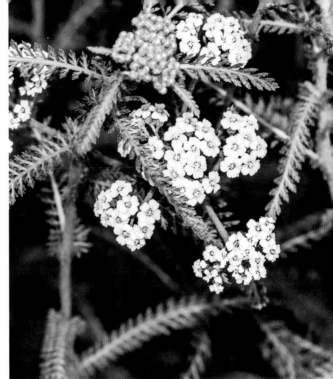
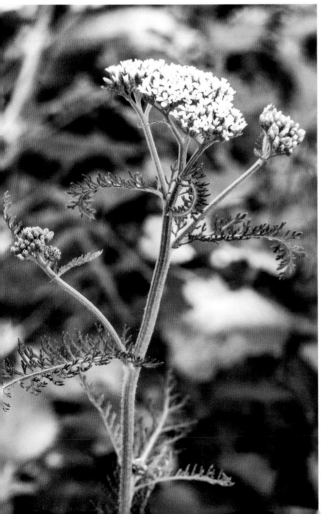

plant and it is quite hardy and easy to establish. When I travelled to the UK I was looking for my beloved herbs and there was Yarrow growing in everyone's lawn. Indicates soil very low in calcium and phosphate and very high in potassium, magnesium and other minerals. Low humus and bacteria with aluminum present.[8]

FURTHER READING Ethnobotany and phytochemistry of yarrow, *Achillea millefolium*, Compositae.[224] In vitro estrogenic activity of *Achillea millefolium* L.[225]

YELLOW DOCK

Curled Dock

Rumex crispus

DISTRIBUTION Native to North Africa and Eurasia and now the most widespread Dock in temperate and subtropical regions. Naturalized throughout Australia mainly in the south-eastern and south-western regions and Tasmania.

HABITAT Common weed in damp soils and drains. Weed of crops, fallows, pastures, waterways and waste areas. Avoids poor soils.

DESCRIPTION

Perennial plant 0.5–1.5 m(1 ft 6 in–5 ft) tall with a distinctive yellow root when scraped.

LEAVES Basal rosette of large, curly leaves and as flowering stem grows the leaves have a 'wrap-around' sheathing on the stem with smaller, narrower leaves.

FLOWERS Large, flowering heads made up of small flowers, which are green when young and reddish-brown as matures. Flowering mostly in the warmer months.

FRUIT/SEED Small, burr-like winged fruits.

USES

EDIBLE/OTHER Leaves, stems and seeds eaten worldwide. Use leaves before flowering, boil in several lots of water then add to soups, pies and stews. Excellent spinach substitute. My favorite is the stems picked before flowering and used to replace rhubarb. I make a delicious Dock and apple crumble. Seeds are edible (related to buckwheat) and have been found in ancient man. American Indians used the ground seeds to make a flour they used in times of famine. One plant can produce 60,000 seeds and they stay viable for 80 years. Collect the seeds when brown (mature). These seeds will contain chaff, which is an insoluble fiber and can act as an irritating bowel cleanser. Remove chaff by winnowing. Use ground in crackers, bread and other dishes. High in Vitamin A, C, calcium, phosphorus and iron. Don't collect Yellow Dock growing in or near drains (contaminants).

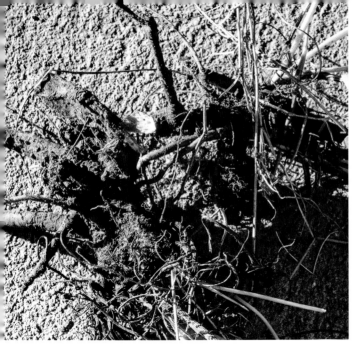

MEDICINAL The yellow root used as a decoction, poultice, tincture, extract or syrup. Used principally as a 'blood cleanser' being effective for skin problems such as dermatitis and psoriasis as well as gently stimulating the bowel. I make a laxative syrup, which achieves good results. High in iron, an excellent tonic, it also aids the liver by stimulating the bile helping with jaundice and other liver complaints. Also used for rheumatism, osteoarthritis and rheumatoid arthritis. A green leaf poultice is used to draw out pus. The cooling oxalates in dock leaves soothe stinging nettle and ant bites.

FARM/ENVIR. Farmers dislike this plant as it reduces grazing capacity but they should be aware that stock usually avoid the leaves and the grasses that grow in sour soil. Docks presence indicates sour, acidic soil, high in moisture and compaction. This plant with its deep taproot is trying to improve the soil taking up the moisture. Eradicate by aerating soils to get rid of damp areas and use humus and lime. Birds enjoy the seeds. Indicates soil low in calcium, very high in phosphate, potassium and magnesium and other minerals. Also high salt, hardpan and with poor drainage.[8]

MAY BE CONFUSED WITH Worldwide there are almost 200 Docks and many are edible although most taste inedible. Yellow Dock is one of the most versatile docks. Broad Leaf Dock (*R. obtusifolius*) is an important weed in Europe and America similar to Yellow Dock however the flower clusters are closer together and plant is larger and spreading. Clustered Dock (*R. conglomeratus*) is a taller dock with flower clusters distant forming a loose leafy pinnacle and valves oblong, blunt and usually with a large swelling.

FURTHER READING Determination of antioxidant and antimicrobial activities of *Rumex crispus* L. extracts.[226]

WARNING High oxalate content. Fatal poisoning by *Rumex crispus* (curled dock): pathological findings and application of scanning electron microscopy.[227]

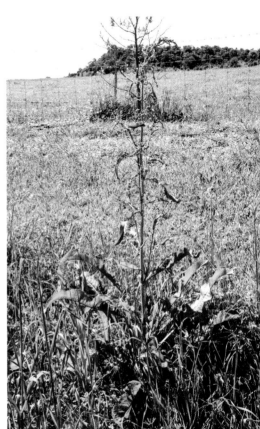

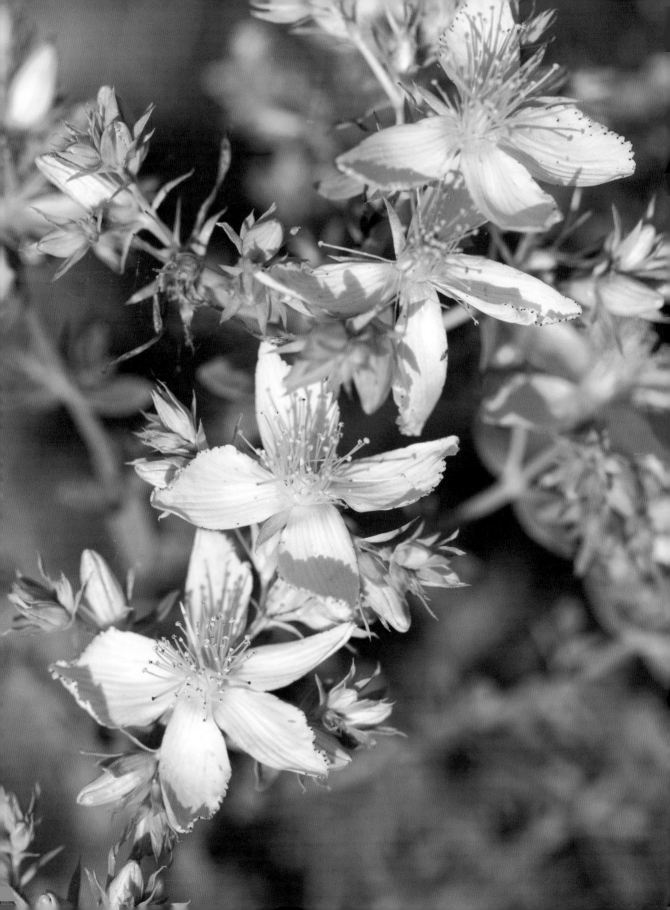

Endnotes

1   Margaret Roberts, *Indigenous Healing Plants*, Southern Book Publishers Pty Ltd, 1990, pp. 5–6.

2   G Krishnamurthy, K Lakshman, N Pruthvi & PU Chandrika, 'Antihyperglycemic and hypolipidemic activity of methanolic extract of Amaranthus viridis leaves in experimental diabetes', *Indian Journal of Pharmacology*, vol. 43(4) Jul–Aug, 2011.

3   G Corea, E Fattorusso & V Lanzotti, 'Saponins and flavonoids of Allium triquetrum', *Journal of Natural Products*, vol. 66(11) Nov, 2003, pp. 1405–11.

4   I Ramírez-Erosa I, Y Huang, RA Hickie et al., 'Xanthatin and xanthinosin from the burs of Xanthium strumarium L. as potential anticancer agents' *Canadian Journal of Physiology and Pharmacoogyl*, vol. 85(11), 2007, pp. 1160–72.

5   B Lin, Y Zhao, P Han et al., 'Anti-arthritic activity of Xanthium strumarium L. extract on complete Freund's adjuvant induced arthritis in rats', *Journal of Ethnopharmacology*, vol. 155 (1), 2014, pp. 248–255.

6   S Tennyson, KJ Ravindran, A Eapen & SJ William, 'Effect of Ageratum houstonianum Mill. (Asteraceae) leaf extracts on the oviposition activity of Anopheles stephensi, Aedes aegypti and Culex quinquefasciatus (Diptera: Culicidae)', *Parasitology Research*, vol. 111(6), 2012, pp. 2295–2299.

6a   S Parveen, R Godara, R Katoch et al., 'In Vitro Evaluation of Ethanolic Extracts of Ageratum conyzoides and Artemisia absinthium against Cattle Tick, Rhipicephalus microplus,' *The Scientific World Journal*, 2014; Srinivas, Reddy et al., *Journal of Advanced Scientific Research*, vol. 3(2), 2012, pp. 67–70.

7   A L Okunade, 'Ageratum conyzoides L. (Asteraceae)', *Fitoterapia*, vol. 73(1) Feb, 2002, pp. 1–16.

8   JL McCaman, 'Weeds and Why they Grow', self-published, Sand Lake USA, 1994, pp. 45–94.

9   YA Abusamra, M Scuruchi, S Habibatni et al., *Pakistan Journal of Pharmaceutical Sciences*, 'Evaluation of putative cytotoxic activity of crude extracts from Onopordum acanthium leaves and Spartium junceum flowers against the U-373 glioblastoma cell line', vol. 28(4), 2015, pp. 1225–32.

10   P Denev, M Kratchanova, M Ciz et al., 'Antioxidant, antimicrobial and neutrophil-modulating activities of herb extracts' *Acta Biochimica Polonica*, vol. 61(2), 2014, pp. 359–67.

10a   V Rameshwar, G Tushar, P Rakesh & G Chetan, 'Rubus fruticosus (blackberry) use as an herbal medicine', *Pharmacognosy Review*, vol. 8(16), 2014, pp. 101–104.

11   RJ Danaher, C Wang, J Dai et al., 'Antiviral Effects of Blackberry Extract Against Herpes Simplex Virus Type 1, *Oral Surgery Oral Medicine Oral Pathology Oral Radiology and Endododontology*, vol. 112(3), 2011.

12   R Gabrani, J Ramya, A Sharma et al., 'Antiproliferative Effect of Solanum nigrum on Human Leukemic Cell Lines', *Indian Journal of Pharmaceutical Sciences*, vol. 74(5), 2012, pp. 451–453.

13 AH Ahmed, IH Kamal & RM Ramzy, 'Studies on the molluscicidal and larvicidal properties of Solanum nigrum L. leaves ethanol extract', *Journal of the Egyptian Society of Parasitology*, vol. 31(3), 2001, pp. 843–52.

14 SK Ahsan, M Tabiq, AM Ageel et al., 'Effect of Trigonella foenum-graecum and Ammi majus on calcium oxalate urolithiasis in rats', *Journal of Ethnopharmacology*, vol. 26 (3), 1989, pp. 249–254.

15 F Ghahremanitamadon, S Shahidi, S Zargooshnia et al., 'Protective Effects of Borago Officinalis Extract On Amyloid Ð-Peptide(25–35) – Induced Memory Impairment In Male Rats: A Behavioral Study', *BioMed Research International*, 2014, pp. 1–8.

16 U Quattrocchi, *CRC World Dictionary of Medicinal and PoisonousPplants: Common Names, Scientific Names, Eponyms, Synonyms, and Stymology*, CRC Press, Boca Raton, FLA, pp. 624–625.

17 K Faidi, N Baaka, S Hammami et al., 'Extraction of carotenoids from Lycium ferocissimum fruits for cotton dyeing: Optimization survey based on a central composite design method', *Fibers and Polymers*, 17(1), 2016, pp. 36–43.

18 Unites States Forest service plants database www.fs.fed.us/database/feis/plants/fern/pteaqu/all.html

19 Herbiguide website www.herbiguide.com.au/Descriptions/hg_Common_Bracken.htm

20 BD Caniceiro, AO Latorre, H Fukumasu et al., 'Immunosuppressive effects of Pteridium aquilinum enhance susceptibility to urethane-induced lung carcinogenesis', *Journal Immunotoxicology*, vol. 12(1), 2015, pp. 74–80.

21 SP Yadav, V Vats, AC Ammini & JK Grover, 'Brassica juncea (Rai) significantly prevented the development of insulin resistance in rats fed fructose-enriched diet', *Journal of Ethnopharmacology*, vol. 93(1) 2004, pp. 113–6.

22 ZH Israili and B Lyoussi, 'Ethnopharmacology of the plants of genus Ajuga', *Pakistan Journal of Pharmaceutical Sciences*, vol. 22(4), 2009, pp.425–462.

23 CABI International Invasive Species Compendium, Typha domingensis (southern cattail) www.cabi.org/isc/datasheet/54296

24 YL Li, YG Liu, JL Liu et al., 'Effects of EDTA on lead uptake by Typha orientalis Presl: a new lead-accumulating species in southern China, *Bulletin of Environmental Contamination and Toxicology*, vol. 81(1), 2008, pp. 36–41.

25 MM Mufarrege, HR Hadad, GA Di Luca & MA Maine, 'The ability of Typha domingensis to accumulate and tolerate high concentrations of Cr, Ni, and Zn', *Environmental Science and Pollution Research International*, vol. 22(1), 2015, pp. 286–92.

26 CC Lin, JM Lu, JJ Yang et al., 'Anti-inflammatory and radical scavenge effects of Arctium lappa', *The American Journal of Chinese Medicine*, vol. 24(2), 1996, pp. 127–37.

27 SC Lin, CH Lin, CC Lin et al., 'Hepatoprotective effects of Arctium lappa Linne on liver injuries induced by chronic ethanol consumption and potentiated by carbon tetrachloride' Journal of Biomedical Science, vol. 9(5), 2002, pp.401–9.

28 O Rop, J Mlcek, T Jurikova et al., 'Edible Flowers—A New Promising Source of Mineral Elements in Human Nutrition', *Molecules*, vol. 17(12), (2012), pp.6672–6683.

29 J-L Wei, H-Y Lai, & Z-S Chen, 'Chelator effects on bioconcentration and translocation of cadmium by hyperaccumulators, Tagetes patula and Impatiens walleriana', *Ecotoxicology and Environmental Safety*, vol. 84, (2012), pp. 173–178.

30 A Rolland, J Fleurentin, MC Lanhers et al., 'Behavioural effects of the American traditional plant Eschscholzia californica: sedative and anxiolytic properties', *Planta Medica,* vol. 57(3), 1991, pp. 212–6.

31 MI Calvo, 'Anti-inflammatory and analgesic activity of the topical preparation of Verbena officinalis L.', *Journal of Ethnopharmacology,* vol. 107(3) 11 Oct, 2006, pp. 380–2. *Journal of Ethnopharmacology,* vol. 7(3) Aug, 2000, pp. 465–72.

32 S Singh, N Vinod & GK Yogendra, 'Evaluation of The Aphrodisiac Activity of Tribulus Terrestris Linn. in Sexually Sluggish Male Albino Rats', *Journal of Pharmacology and Pharmacotherapeutics,* vol. 3(1), 2012.

33 K Gauthaman & AP Ganesan, 'The hormonal effects of Tribulus terrestris and its role in the management of male erectile dysfunction – an evaluation using primates, rabbit and rat', *Phytomedicine,* vol. 15(1–2), 2008, pp. 44–54.

34 S Ojha, M Nandave, S Arora et al., 'Chronic Administration of Tribulus terrestris Linn. Extract Improves Cardiac Function and Attenuates Myocardial Infarction in Rats', *International Journal of Pharmacology,* vol. 4(1), 2008, pp. 1–10.

35 M Haloui, L Louedec, JB Michel & B Lyoussi, 'Experimental diuretic effects of Rosmarinus officinalis and Centaurium erythraea', *Journal of Ethnopharmacology,* vol. 71(3), 2000, pp. 465–472.

36 M Mroueh, Y Saab & R Rizkallah, 'Hepatoprotective activity of Centaurium erythraea on acetaminophen-induced hepatotoxicity in rats', *Phytotherapy Research,* vol. 18(5), 2004, pp. 431–433.

37 P Valentao, E Fernandes, F Carvalho et al., 'Antioxidant activity of Centaurium erythraea infusion evidenced by its superoxide radical scavenging and xanthine oxidase inhibitory activity', *Journal of Agricultural and Food Chemistry,* vol. 49(7), 2001, pp. 3476–3479.

38 N Rani, N Vasudeva & SK Sharma, 'Quality assessment and anti-obesity activity of Stellaria media (Linn.) Vill', *BMC Complementary Alternative Medicine,* vol. 12(145), 2012.

39 L Ma, J Song, Y Shi et al., 'Anti-Hepatitis B Virus Activity of Chickweed [Stellaria Media (L.) Vill.] Extracts In HepG2.2.15 Cells', *Molecules,* vol. 17(7), 2012, pp. 8633–8646.

40 EA Rogozhin, MP Slezina, AA Slavokhotova et al., 'A Novel Antifungal Peptide from Leaves of The Weed Stellaria Media L', *Biochimie,* vol. 116.2015, pp. 125–132.

41 DG Sobey, 'Stellaria Media (L.) Vill.', *The Journal of Ecology,* vol. 69(1), 1981.

42 RA Street, S Jasmeen & G Prinsloo, 'Cichorium Intybus: Traditional Uses, Phytochemistry, Pharmacology, and Toxicology', *Evidence-Based Complementary and Alternative Medicine,* 2013, pp. 1–13.

43 J Bokhari, MR Khan, M Shabbir et al., 'Evaluation of Diverse Antioxidant Activities of Galium Aparine', *Spectrochimica acta Part A: Molecular and Biomolecular Spectroscopy,* vol. 102, 2013, pp. 24–29.

44 FJB Quinlan, 'Galium Aparine As A Remedy For Chronic Ulcers', *The British Medical Journal,* vol. 1 (1172), 1883, pp. 1173–1174.

45 V Tangpu, K Temjenmongla & AK Yadav, 'Anticestodal Activity of Trifolium repens. Extract.', *Pharmaceutical Biology,* vol. 42(8), 2005, pp. 656–658.

46 Office of the Gene Technology Regulator, 'The Biology and Ecology of White Clover (Trifolium repens L.) in Australia', July 2004, www.ogtr.gov.au/internet/ogtr/publishing.nsf/content/clover-3/$FILE/biologywclover 2.pdf.

47 AP Bartolome, IM Villaseñor, and W-C Yang, 'Bidens Pilosal. (Asteraceae): Botanical Properties, Traditional Uses, Phytochemistry, and Pharmacology', *Evidence-Based Complementary and Alternative Medicine*, vol. 2013(2), pp. 1–51.

48 MG Brandão, AU Krettli, LS Soares et al., 'Antimalarial Activity of Extracts and Fractions From Bidens Pilosa and Other Bidens Species (Asteraceae) Correlated with The Presence of Acetylene and Flavonoid Compounds', *Journal of Ethnopharmacology*, vol. 57(2), 1997, pp. 131–138.

49 BA Clare, RS Conroy & K Spelman, 'The Diuretic Effect In Human Subjects of An Extract of Taraxacum Officinale Folium Over A Single Day', *The Journal of Alternative and Complementary Medicine*, vol. 15(8), 2009, pp. 929–934.

50 Y-J Koh, DS Cha, JS Ko et al., 'Anti-Inflammatory Effect of Taraxacum Officinale Leaves On Lipopolysaccharide-Induced Inflammatory Responses In RAW 264.7 Cells', *Journal of Medicinal Food*, vol. 13(4), 2010, pp. 870–878.

51 U-K Choi, O-H Lee, J-H Yim et al., 'Hypolipidemic and Antioxidant Effects of Dandelion (Taraxacum Officinale) Root and Leaf On Cholesterol-Fed Rabbits', *International Journal of Molecular Sciences*, vol. 11(1), 2010, pp. 67–87.

52 Y Yang & S Li, 'Dandelion Extracts Protect Human Skin Fibroblasts From UVB Damage and Cellular Senescence', *Oxidative Medicine and Cellular Longevity*, 2015, pp. 1–10.

53 J Janick & A Whipkey, *Issues In New Crops and New Uses*, ASHA Press, Alexandria, VA, 2007, pp. 284–292.

54 V Schmitzer, R Veberic, A Slatnar & F Stampar, 'Elderberry (Sambucus Nigra L.) Wine: A Product Rich In Health Promoting Compounds', *Journal of Agricultural and Food Chemistry*, vol. 58(18), 2010, pp. 10143–10146.

55 A Olejnik, M Olkowicz, K Kowalska et al., 'Gastrointestinal Digested Sambucus Nigra L. Fruit Extract Protects In Vitro Cultured Human Colon Cells Against Oxidative Stress', *Food Chemistry*, vol. 197(Part A), 2016, pp. 648–657.

56 FP Karakaş, A Karakaş, Ç Boran et al., 'The evaluation of topical administration of Bellis perennis fraction on circular excision wound healing in Wistar albino rats', *Pharmaceutical Biology*, vol. 50(8), 2012.

57 FP Karakaş, A Karakaş, H Coskun & AC Türker, 'Effects of common daisy (Bellis perennis L.) aqueous extracts on anxiety-like behaviour and spatial memory performance in Wistar albino rats', *African Journal of Pharmacy and Pharmacology*, vol. 5(11), 2011, pp.1378–1388.

58 J Senguttuvan, P Subramaniam & K Krishnamoorthy Karthika, 'Phytochemical Analysis and Evaluation of Leaf and Root Parts of The Medicinal Herb, Hypochaeris Radicata L. For In Vitro Antioxidant Activities', *Asian Pacific Journal of Tropical Biomedicine*, vol. 4 (Suppl. 1), 2014: S359–S367.

59 S Jamuna, S Paulsamy & K Karthika, 'In-vitro antibacterial activity of leaf and root extracts of Hypochaeris Radicata L. (Asteraceae) – a medicinal plant species inhabiting the high hills of Nilgiris, the western Ghats, '*International Journal of Pharmacy and Pharmaceutical Sciences*, vol. 5(1), 2013.

60 A Jabbar, MA Zaman, Z Iqbal et al., 'Anthelmintic activity of Chenopodium album (L.) and Caesalpinia crista (L.) against trichostrongylid nematodes of sheep', *Journal of Ethnopharmacology*, vol. 114(1), 2007, pp. 86–91. M Khoobchandani, BK Ojeswi, B Sharma & MM Srivastava, MM. 'Chenopodium album prevents progression of cell growth and enhances cell toxicity in human breast cancer cell lines', *Oxidative Medicine and Cellular Longevity*, vol, 2(3) July–Aug, 2009, pp. 160–165.

61 K Bone & S Mills, *Principles and Practice of Phytotherapy: Modern Herbal Medicine*, Churchill Livingstone, UK, 2012, pp. 560–562.

62 K Javidnia, L Dastgheib, SM Samani & A Nasiri, 'Antihirsutism activity of fennel (fruits of Foeniculum vulgare) extract–a double-blind placebo controlled study', *Phytomedicine*, vol. 10(6), 2003, pp.455–458.

63 E Ernst & MH Pittler, 'The efficacy and safety of feverfew (Tanacetum parthenium L.): an update of a systematic review', *Public health nutrition*, vol. 3(4a), 2000, pp. 509–514.

64 JP Blakeman & P Atkinson, 'Antimicrobial properties and possible role in host-pathogen interactions of parthenolide, a sesquiterpene lactone isolated from glands of Chrysanthemum parthenium', *Physiological Plant Pathology*, vol. 15(2), 1979, pp. 183–192.

65 A Pareek, M Suthar, GS Rathore & V Bansal, 'Feverfew (Tanacetum parthenium L.): A systematic review', *Pharmacognosy Reviews*, vol. 5(9), 2011, pp. 103–110.

66 AG Kachenko, B Singh & NP Bhatia, 'Heavy metal tolerance in common fern species', *Australian Journal of Botany*, vol. 55(1), 2007.

66 A Aksoy, WH Hale, JM Dixon, 'Capsella bursa-pastoris (L.) Medic. as a biomonitor of heavy metals', *Science of The Total Environment*, vol. 226(2–3), 1999, pp. 177–186.

67 PK Dantu, R Dolly & PB Khare, 'In Vitro Antibacterial and Antifungal Properties of Aqueous and Non-Aqueous Frond Extracts of Psilotum Nudum, Nephrolepis Biserrata and Nephrolepis Cordifolia', *Indian Journal of Pharmaceutical Sciences*, vol. 72(6), 2010.

68 U Quattrocchi, *CRC world dictionary of medicinal and poisonous plants: Common names, scientific names, eponyms, synonyms, and etymology*, CRC Press, Boca Raton, FLA, 2012.

69 YA Abusamra, M Scuruchi, S Habibatni et al., 'Evaluation of putative cytotoxic activity of crude extracts from Onopordum acanthium leaves and Spartium junceum flowers against the U-373 glioblastoma cell line', *Pakistan Journal of Pharmaceutical Sciences*, vol. 1(28), 2015, pp. 1225–1232.

70 IA Bukhari, AJ Shah, RA Khan et al., 'Gut modulator effects of Conyza bonariensis explain its traditional use in constipation and diarrhea', *European Review for Medical and Pharmacological Sciences*, vol. 17(4), 2013. p. 552.

71 Rain-tree.com Tropical Plant Database last updated 28/12/2012 www.rain-tree.com/clavillia.htm#.Vv8jrjx95pg

72 A Maxia, C Sanna, B Salve et al., 'Inhibition of Histamine Mediated Responses By Mirabilis Jalapa : Confirming Traditional Claims Made About Antiallergic and Antiasthmatic Activity' *Natural Product Research*, vol. 24(18), 2010, pp. 1681–1686.

73 M Singh, V Kumar, I Singh et al., 'Anti-Inflammatory Activity of Aqueous Extract of Mirabilis Jalapa Linn. Leaves', *Pharmacognosy Research*, vol. 2(6), 2010.

74 J Soušek, C Vavrecková, J Psotová et al., 'Antioxidant and antilipoperoxidant activities of alkaloid and phenolic extracts of eight fumaria species', *Acta Horticulturae*, vol. 501, 1999, pp. 239–244.

74a GH Schmelzer & A Gurib-Fakim (eds.), *Medicinal Plants 1 Plant Resources of Tropical Africa*, Prota Foundation, 2008.

75 United States Dept of Agriculture Natural Resources Conservation Service Plant Guide, prepared by Pamela LS Pavek, published 9/2011 plants.usda.gov/plantguide/pdf/pg_soca6.pdf.

76 P Apáti P, PJ Houghton & A Kéry, 'HPLC investigation of antioxidant components in Solidago herba', *Acta Pharmaceutica Hungarica*, vol. 74(4), 2004, pp. 223–231.

77 Cabi.org Invasive Species Compendium www.cabi.org/isc/datasheet/16496 Updated 11/1/08 by Nick Pasiecznik, consultant, France.

78 K Bone & S Mills, *Principles and Practice of Phytotherapy*, 2nd edition, Churchill Livingstone (Elsevier), 2013, pp. 671–684.

79 S Rimkiene, O Ragazinskiene & N Savickiene, 'The cumulation of Wild pansy (Viola tricolor L.) accessions: the possibility of species preservation and usage in medicine', *Medicina (Kaunas)*, vol. 39(4), 2003, pp. 411–416.

80 R Hellinger, J Koehbach, H Fedchuk et al., 'Immunosuppressive Activity of An Aqueous Viola Tricolor Herbal Extract', *Journal of Ethnopharmacology*, vol. 151(1), 2014, pp. 299–306.

80a RAS Thabit, XR Cheng, X Tang et al., 'Antioxidant and antibacterial activities of extracts from Conyza bonariensis growing in Yemen', *Pakistan Journal of Pharmaceutical Sciences*, vol. 28(1), 2015, pp.129–134.

81 A Di Sotto, A Vitalone, M Nicoletti et al., 'Pharmacological and phytochemical study on a Sisymbrium officinale Scop. extract', *Journal of Ethnopharmacology*, vol. 127(3), 2010, pp. 731–736. CABI International Invasive Species Compendium, 'Typha domingensis (southern cattail)', www.cabi.org/isc/datasheet/54296.

82 A Jabbar, MA Raza, Z Iqbal & MN Khan, 'An inventory of the ethnobotanicals used as anthelmintics in the southern Punjab (Pakistan)', *Journal of Ethnopharmacology*, 108(1), 2006, pp. 152–154.

83 SE Sajjadi & A Ghannadi, 'Analysis of the Essential Oil of Lamium amplexicaule L. from Northeastern Iran', *Journal of Essential Oil Bearing Plants*, vol. 15(4), 2012, pp. 577–581.

84 U Quattrocchi, *CRC world dictionary of medicinal and poisonous plants: Common names, scientific names, eponyms, synonyms, and etymology*, CRC Press, Boca Raton, FLA, 2012.

85 Weeds of Australia Biosecurity Queensland Edition, Fact Sheet, keyserver.lucidcentral.org/weeds/data/media/Html/gleditsia_triacanthos.htm

86 M Üner & T Altınkurt, 'Evaluation of Honey Locust (Gleditsia Triacanthos Linn.) Gum As Sustaining Material In Tablet Dosage Forms', *Il Farmaco*, vol. 59(7), 2004, pp. 567–573.

87 DO Saleh, I Kassem & and FR Melek, 'Analgesic Activity of Gleditsia Triacanthos Methanolic Fruit Extract and Its Saponin-Containing Fraction', *Pharmaceutical Biology*, vol. 54(4), 2015, pp. 576–580.

88 JH Lee, WS Ko, YH Kim et al., 'Anti-inflammatory effect of the aqueous extract from Lonicera japonica flower is related to inhibition of NF-kappaB activation through reducing

I-kappaBalpha degradation in rat liver', *International Journal of Molecular Medicine*, vol. 7(1), 2001, pp. 79–83.

89   TF Tzeng, SS Liou, CJ Chang & IM Liu, 'The Ethanol Extract of Lonicera Japonica (Japanese Honeysuckle) Attenuates Diabetic Nephropathy By Inhibiting P-38 MAPK Activity In Streptozotocin-Induced Diabetic Rats', *Planta Medica*, vol. 80(2–3), 2014, pp. 121–129.

90   H-J Yoo, HJ Kang, YS Song et al., 'Anti-Angiogenic, Antinociceptive and Anti-Inflammatory Activities of Lonicera Japonica Extract', *Journal of Pharmacy and Pharmacology*, vol. 60(6), 2008, pp. 779–786.

90a Bush craft, Edible Wild Plants Survival tips, Wilderness Survival Internet 2016 blog. emergencyoutdoors.com/edible-wild-plants-japanese-honeysuckle-lonicera-japonica/

91   S El Bardai, B Lyoussi, M Wibo, N Morel, 'Comparative study of the antihypertensive activity of Marrubium vulgare and of the dihydropyridine calcium antagonist amlodipine in spontaneously hypertensive rat', *Clinical and Experimental Hypertension*, vol. 26(6), 2004, pp. 465–74.

92   C Meyre-Silva, RA Yunes, V Schlemper et al., 'Analgesic potential of marrubiin derivatives, a bioactive diterpene present in Marrubium vulgare (Lamiaceae)', *Farmaco*, vol. 60(4), 2005, pp. 321–326.

93   R Manivannan & S Ilayaraja, 'Kaempferol-3-O-Ð-L-Arabinopyranosyl(1Ð6)-Ð-D-Galactopyranoside From Phytolacca Octandra and Its Antimicrobial Activity', *Chemistry of Natural Compounds*, vol. 49(2), 2013, pp. 336–337.

94   RJ Grayer & JB Harborne, 'A survey of antifungal compounds from higher plants, 1982–1993', *Phytochemistry*, vol. 37(1), 1994, pp. 19–42.

95   LA Al-Shammari, WH Hassan & HM Al-Youssef, 'Phytochemical and biological studies of Carduus pycnocephalus L.', *Journal of Saudi Chemical Society*, vol. 19(4), 2015, pp. 410–416.

96   'Jasmine (Jasminum spp.)', www.westerlynaturalmarket.com/ns/DisplayMonograph.asp?-StoreID=qwcsn3n89asr2js000akhmccqab04fn2&DocID=bottomline-jasmine

97   WC Chang, H Jia, W Aw, et al., 'Beneficial Effects of Soluble Dietary Jerusalem Artichoke (Helianthus Tuberosus) In The Prevention of The Onset of Type 2 Diabetes and Non-Alcoholic Fatty Liver Disease In High-Fructose Diet-Fed Rats', *British Journal of Nutrition*, vol. 112(5), 2014, pp. 709–717.

98   JL Kim, CR Bae & YS Cha, 'Helianthus tuberosus Extract Has Anti-Diabetes Effects in HIT-T15 Cells', *Food and Agriculture Organization of the United Nation Agris*, Jan 2010.

99   Y-Y Sung, T Yoon, W-K Yang et al., 'The Antiobesity Effect of Polygonum Aviculare L. Ethanol Extract In High-Fat Diet-Induced Obese Mice', *Evidence-Based Complementary and Alternative Medicine*, 2013, pp. 1–11.

100 CY Hsu, 'Antioxidant activity of extract from Polygonum aviculare L.', *Biological Research*, vol, 39(2), 2006, pp. 281–8.

101 VK Dua, NC Gupta, AC Pandey & VP Sharma, 'Repellency of Lantana Camara (verbenaceae) flowers against Aedes mosquitoes', *Journal of the American Mosquito Control Association*, vol 12 (3 Pt 1), 1996, pp. 406–408.

102 VK Dua, AC Pandey & AP Dash, 'Adultical activity of essential oil of Lantana camara leaves against mosquitoes', *Indian Journal of Medical Research*, vol. 131, 2010, pp. 434–439.

103 F Barreto, E Soussa, A Campos, et al., 'Antibacterial Activity of Lantana Camara Linn Lantana Montevidensis Brig Extracts From Cariri-Ceara, Brazil'. *Journal of Young Pharmacists*, vol. 2(1), 2010, pp. 42–44.

104 N Mimica-Dukic, B Bozin, M Sokovic & N Simin, 'Antimicrobial and antioxidant activities of Melissa officinalis L.(Lamiaceae) essential oil', *Journal of agricultural and food chemistry*, vol. 52(9), 2004, pp.2485–2489.

105 A Akhondzadeh, 'Melissa officinalis extract in the treatment of patients with mild to moderate Alzheimer's disease: a double blind, randomised, placebo controlled trial', *Journal of Neurology, Neurosurgery & Psychiatry*, vol. 74(7), 2003, pp. 863–866.

106 RH Wölbling, & K Leonhardt, 'Local therapy of herpes simplex with dried extract from Melissa officinalis', *Phytomedicine*, vol. 1(1), 1994, pp. 25–31.

107 'L-Canavanine', www.uky.edu/~garose/cav2.htm.

108 KS Bora & A Sharma, 'Evaluation of Antioxidant and Cerebroprotective Effect of Medicago Sativa Linn. Against Ischemia and Repefushion Insult', *Evidence-Based Complementary & Alternative Medicine*, 2011.

109 TL Shale, WA Stirk & J van Staden, 'Variation in antibacterial and anti-inflammatory activity of different growth forms of Malva Parviflora and evidence for synergism of anti-inflammatory compounds', *Journal of Ethnopharmacology*, vol. 96(1–2), 2005.

110 AG Filho, 'Biological Activity of Secondary Metabolites of Buddleja brasiliensis and Artemisia Verlotorm', Federal University of De Santa Maria, 2011. cascavel.ufsm.br/tede//tde_busca/arquivo.php?codArquivo=4802

111 LF Bittencourt De Souza, HD Laughinghouse IV, T Pastori, et al., 'Genotoxic potential of aqueous extracts of Artemisia verlotorum on the cell cycle of Allium cepa', *International Journal of Environmental Studies*, vol. 67(6), 2010. www.tandfonline.com/doi/abs/10.1080/00207233.2010.520457

112 L Braun, & M Cohen, *Herbs & natural supplements an evidence-based guide volume 2*, 4th edition, Churchill Livingstone (Elsevier), pp. 695–697.

113 AU Turker & G Ekrem, 'Common Mullein (Verbascum Thapsus L.): Recent Advances In Research', *Phytotherapy Research*, vol. 19(9), 2005, pp.733–739.

114 N Ali, SW Ali Shah, I Shah et al., 'Anthelmintic and Relaxant Activities of Verbascum Thapsus Mullein', *BMC Complementary and Alternative Medicine*, vol. 12(1), 2012.

115 R Mandera & U Meyer, 'Portrait of a Medicinal Plant—Tropaeolum Majus—Nasturtium', *Journal of Anthroposophical Medicine*, vol. 12(4), 1995. (www.anthromed.org/Article.aspx?artpk=248)

116 A Gasparotto, GM Gasparotto, EL Lourenço et al., 'Antihypertensive Effects of Isoquercitrin and Extracts From Tropaeolum Majus L.: Evidence For The Inhibition of Angiotensin Converting Enzyme', *Journal of Ethnopharmacology*, vol. 134(2), 2011, pp. 363–372.

117 C Gomes, EL Lourenço, EB Liuti et al., 'Evaluation of subchronic toxicity of the hydro-ethanolic extract of Tropaeolum majus in Wistar rats', *Journal of Ethnopharmacology*, vol. 142(2), 2012, pp. 481–487. (www.sciencedirect.com/science/article/pii/S0378874112003339)

118 K Bone & S Mills, *Nettle (Urtica Dioica L. Urtic urens L.) Principles and Practice of Phytotherapy: Modern Herbal Medicine*, 2nd Edition, Churchill Livingstone (Elsevier), 2013.

119 MR Safarinejad, 'Urtica dioica for treatment of benign prostatic hyperplasia: a prospective, randomized, double-blind, placebo-controlled, crossover study', *Journal of Herbal Pharmacotherapy*, vol. 5(4), 2005, pp. 1–11.

120 M Nassiri-Asl, F Zamansoltani, E Abassi et al., 'Effects of Urtica Dioica Extract On Lipid Profile In Hypercholesterolemic Rats', *Journal of Chinese Integrative Medicine*, vol. 7(5), 2009, pp. 428–433.

121 U Quattrocch, *CRC world dictionary of medicinal and poisonous plants: Common names, scientific names, eponyms, synonyms, and etymology*, CRC Press, Boca Raton, FLA, 2012.

122 Maiden, JH, *The weeds of New South Wales part 1*, Government Printer, Sydney, 1920, pp. 98–104.

123 I Ramírez-Erosa, Y Huang, RA Hickie et al., 'Xanthatin and Xanthinosin From The Burs of Xanthium Strumarium L. As Potential Anticancer Agents', *Canadian Journal of Physiology and Pharmacology*, vol. 85(11), 2007, pp. 1160–1172.

124 L-M Xue, QY Zhang, P Han et al., 'Hepatotoxic Constituents and Toxicological Mechanism of Xanthium Strumarium L. Fruits', *Journal of Ethnopharmacology*, vol. 152(2), 2014, pp. 272–282.

125 AC Igboasoiyi, OA Eseyin, NK Ezenwa & HO Oladimeji, 'Studies on the Toxicity of Ageratum conyzoides', *Journal of Pharmacology and Toxicology*, vol. 2(8), 2007, pp. 743–747.

126 H Imam, G Sofi, A Seikh & A Lone, 'The incredible benefits of Nagarmotha (Cyperus rotundus)' *International Journal of Nutrition, Pharmacology, Neurological Diseases*, vol. 4(1), 2014, p. 23.

127 NA Raut, NJ Gaikwad, Antidiabetic activity of hydro-ethanolic extract of Cyperus rotundus in alloxan induced diabetes in rats, *Fitoterapia*, vol. 77(7–8), 2006, pp. 585–588.

128 S Kilani, M Ben Sghaier, I Limem et al., 'In vitro evaluation of antibacterial, antioxidant, cytotoxic and apoptotic activities of the tubers infusion and extracts of Cyperus rotundus', *Bioresource Technology*, vol. 99(18), 2008, pp. 9004–9008.

129 AH Ahmed & MM Rifaat 'Molluscicidal and cercaricidal efficacy of Acanthus mollis and its binary and tertiary combinations with Solanum nigrum and Iris pseudacorus against Biomphalaria alexandrina', *Journal of the Egyptian Society of Parasitology*, vol. 34(3), 2004, pp. 1041–1050.

130 U Quattrocchi, *CRC world dictionary of medicinal and poisonous plants: Common names, scientific names, eponyms, synonyms, and etymology*, CRC Press, Boca Raton, FLA, 2012.

131 RT Narendhirakannan & TP Limmy, 'Anti-Inflammatory and Anti-Oxidant Properties of Sida Rhombifolia Stems and Roots In Adjuvant Induced Arthritic Rats', *Immunopharmacology and Immunotoxicology*, vol. 34(2), 2011, pp. 326–336.

132 ME Islam, ME Haque & MA Mosaddik, 'Cytotoxicity and Antibacterial Activity Ofsida Rhombifolia (Malvaceae) Grown In Bangladesh', *Phytotherapy Research*, vol. 17(8), 2003, pp. 973–975.

133 SR Gupta, SA Nirmal, RY Patil & GS Asane, 'Anti-Arthritic Activity of Various Extracts of Sida Rhombifolia Aerial Parts', *Natural Product Research*, vol. 23(8), 2009, pp. 689–695.

134 RE Uncinci Manganelli, L Zaccaro & PE Tomei, 'Antiviral activity in vitro of Urtica dioica L., Parietaria diffusa M. et K. and Sambucus nigra L.', *Journal of Ethnopharmacology*, vol. 98(3), 2005, pp. 323–327.

135 E Yarnell, 'Botanical Medicines for the Urinary Tract', *World Journal of Urology*, vol. 20(5), 2002, pp. 285–293.

136 KJ Gohil, JA Patel & AK Gajjar, 'Pharmacological Review On Centella Asiatica: A Potential Herbal Cure-All', *Indian Journal of Pharmaceutical Sciences,* vol. 72(5), 2010, pp. 546–556.

137 Useful Tropical Plants Database 2014, tropical.theferns.info/viewtropical.php?id=Schinus+molle

138 H Bendaoud, M Romdhane, JP Souchard et al,. 'Chemical Composition and Anticancer and Antioxidant Activities of Schinus Molle L. and Schinus Terebinthifolius Raddi Berries Essential Oils', *Journal of Food Science,* vol. 75(6), 2010, pp. C466–C472.

139 E Abdel-Sattar, AA Zitoun, MA Farg et al., 'Chemical Composition, Insecticidal and Insect Repellent Activity of Schinus Molle L. Leaf and Fruit Essential Oils Against Trogoderma Granarium and Tribolium Castaneum', *Natural Product Research,* vol. 24(3), 2010, pp. 226–235.

140 M van de Venter, S Roux, LC Bungu et al., 'Antidiabetic screening and scoring of 11 plants traditionally used in South Africa', *Journal of Ethnopharmacology,* vol. 119(1), 2008, pp. 81–86.

141 'Euphorbia peplus', www.radiumweed.com.au.

142 JR Ramsay, A Suhrbier, JH Aylward et al., 'The Sap From Euphorbia Peplus Is Effective Against Human Nonmelanoma Skin Cancers', *British Journal of Dermatology,* vol. 164(3)

142 'Invasive Species Compendium Tagetes minuta (Stinking roger)', www.cabi.org/isc/datasheet/52642.

143 AV Steward, 'Plantain (Plantago lanceolate) – a potential Pasture Species', *Proceedings of the New Zealand Grassland Association,* vol. 58, 1996, pp. 77–86.

144 AB Samuelsen, The traditional uses, chemical constituents and biological activities of Plantago major L. A review', *Journal of Ethnopharmacology,* vol. 71(1–2), 2000, pp. 1–21.

145 F Baroni, A Boscagli, G Protano & F Riccobono, 'Antimony accumulation in Achillea ageratum, Plantago lanceolata and Silene vulgaris growing in an old Sb-mining area', *Environmental Pollution,* vol. 109(2), 2000. pp. 347–352.

146 S Mifsud, 'Opium poppy (Papaver somniferum spp L.)', Wild Plants of the Mediterranean Islands of Malta, www.maltawildplants.com/PAPV/Papaver_somniferum_subsp_setigerum.php

147 PJ Garnock-Jones, & P Scholes, 'Alkaloid Content of Papaver Somniferum Subsp. Setigerum From New Zealand', *New Zealand Journal of Botany,* vol. 28(3), 1990, pp. 367–369

148 CA Damalas, 'Distribution, biology, and agricultural importance of Galinsoga parviflora (Asteraceae)', *Weed Biology and Management,* vol. 8, 2008, pp. 147–153.

149 L Lin, Q Jin, Y Liu et al., 'Screening of a new cadmium hyperaccumulator, Galinsoga parviflora, from winter farmland weeds using the artificially high soil cadmium concentration method', *Environmental Toxicology and Chemistry,* vol. 33(11), 2014, pp. 2422–2428.

150 KH Janbaz, MF Latif, F Saqib et al., 'Pharmacological Effects of Lactuca serriola L. in Experimental Model of Gastrointestinal, Respiratory, and Vascular Ailments', *Evidence-Based Complementary and Alternative Medicine,* volume 2013, 2013, pp. 1–9.

151 T Low, *Bush Medicine,* Angus & Robertson, North Ryde, NSW, 1990, p. 58.

152 W Xie & L Du, 'Diabetes Is An Inflammatory Disease: Evidence From Traditional Chinese Medicines', *Diabetes, Obesity and Metabolism,* vol. 13(4), 2011, pp. 289–301.

153 S Chauhan, N Sheth, N Jivani et al., 'Biological actions of Opuntia species', *Systematic Reviews in Pharmacy*, vol. 1(2), 2010, p. 146.

154 AB Cowper, *Common medicinal plants of Australia*, Rose Print, Sydney, 1987, pp. 48–50.

155 AP Simopoulos, HA Norman, JE Gillaspy & JA Duke, 'Common purslane: a source of omega-3 fatty acids and antioxidants', *Journal of the American College of Nutrition*, vol. 11(4), 1992, pp. 374–382.

156 AN Rashed, FU Afifi & AM Disi, 'Simple evaluation of the wound healing activity of a crude extract of Portulaca oleracea L. (growing in Jordan) in Mus musculus JVI-1', *Journal of Ethnopharmacology*, vol. 88(2–3), 2003, pp. 131–136.

157 G Schmeda-Hirschmann, J Loyola, J I Sierra et al., 'Hypotensive effect and enzyme inhibition activity of mapuche medicinal plant extracts', *Phytotherapy Research*, vol. 6(4), 1992, pp. 184–188.

158 A Bocheva, B Mikhova, R Taskova et al., 'Antiinflammatory and analgesic effects of Carthamus lanatus aerial parts', *Fitoterapia*, vol. 74(6), 2003, pp. 559–563.

159 C Zidorn, U Lohwasser, S Pschorr et al., 'Bibenzyls and dihydroisocoumarins from white salsify (Tragopogon porrifolius subsp. porrifolius)', *Phytochemistry*, vol. 66(14), 2005, pp. 1691–1697.

160 M Amoros, B Fauconnier & R Girre, 'In vitro antiviral activity of a saponin from Anagallis arvensis, Primulaceae, against herpes simplex virus and poliovirus', *Antiviral Research*, vol. 8(1), 1987, pp. 13–25.

161 YL Nene, & PN Thapliyal, 'Antifungal properties of Anagallis arvensis L. extract. Naturwissenschaften', vol. 52(4), 1965, pp. 89–90.

162 SY Ryu, M-H Oak, S-K Yoon et al., 'Anti-Allergic and Anti-Inflammatory Triterpenes from the Herb of Prunella vulgaris. Planta Medica', vol. 66(4), 2000, pp. 358–360.

163 X-J Yao, MA Wainberg & MA Parniak, 'Mechanism of inhibition of HIV-1 infection in Vitro by purified extract of Prunella vulgaris', *Virology*, vol. 187(1), 1992, pp. 56–62.

164 www.healthfreedom.info/cancer%20essiac.htm

165 L Migliore, C Civitareale, G Brambilla et al., 'Effects of sulphadimethoxine on cosmopolitan weeds (Amaranthus retroflexus L., Plantago major L. and Rumex acetosella L.)', *Agriculture, Ecosystems & Environment*, vol. 65(2), 1997, pp. 163–168.

166 A Aksoy, WH Hale & JM Dixon, 'Capsella bursa-pastoris (L.) Medic. as a biomonitor of heavy metals', *Science of the Total Environment*, vol. 226(2), 1999, pp. 177–186.

167 K Kuroda, M Akao, M Kanisawa & Miyaki, 'Inhibitory effect of Capsella bursa-pastoris extract on growth of Ehrlich solid tumor in mice', *Cancer Research*, vol. 36(6), 1976, pp. 1900–1903.

168 HB Sahoo, DD Santani & R Sagar, 'Chemopreventive potential of Apium leptophyllum (Pers.) against DMBA induced skin carcinogenesis model by modulatory influence on biochemical and antioxidant biomarkers in Swiss mice', *Indian Journal of Pharmacology*, vol. 46(5), 2014, p. 531.

169 earthmedicineinstitute.com/more/library/medicinal-plants/sonchus-oleraceus/

170 JL Guil-Guerrero, A Giménez-Giménez, I Rodríguez-García, & ME Torija-Isasa, 'Nutritional composition of Sonchus species (S asper L., S oleraceus L. and S tenerrimus L.)', *Journal of the Science of Food and Agriculture*, vol. 76(4), 1998, pp. 628–632.

171 F Cardoso Vilela, R Soncini & A Giusti-Paiva, 'Anxiolytic-like effect of Sonchus oleraceus L. in mice', *Journal of Ethnopharmacology*, vol. 124(2), 2009, pp. 325–327.

172 I Saracoglu, & US Harput, 'In Vitro Cytotoxic Activity and Structure Activity Relationships of Iridoid Glucosides Derived from Veronica species', *Phytotherapy Research*, vol. 26(1), 2011, pp. 148–152.

173 US Harput, I Saracoglu, M Inoue & Y Ogihara, 'Phenylethanoid and iridoid glycosides from Veronica persica', *Chemical and Pharmaceutical Bulletin*, vol. 50(6), 2002, pp. 869–871.

174 CAB International Invasive Species Compendium Emex australis (Doublegee) www.cabi.org/isc/datasheet/20826

175 AE Donia, GA Soliman, MA El-Sakhawy et al., 'Cytotoxic and antimicrobial activities of Emex spinosa (L.) Campd. extract', *Pakistan Journal of Pharmaceutical Sciences*, vol. 27(2), 2014, pp. 351–356.

176 MA Grieve, *Modern herbal*, Tiger Books International, London, 1992, first published in 1931 by Jonathan Cape Ltd, pp. 97–99.

177 D Rayburn, *Let's get natural with herbs: the most complete A–Z reference guide to utilizing herbs for health and beauty*, Ozark Mountain Publishing, 2007.

178 JH Maiden, *The weeds of New South Wales part 1*, Government Printer, Sydney, 1920, pp. 72–74.

178a *Weed control using goats*, Meat and Livestock Australia Ltd, 2007.

179 AW Philbey, AM Hawker & JV Evers, 'A Neurological Locomotor Disorder In Sheep Grazing Stachys Arvensis', *Australian Veterinary Journal*, vol. 79(6), 2001, pp. 427–430.

180 ML Tereschuk, MV, Riera, GR Castro & LR Abdala, 'Antimicrobial activity of flavonoids from leaves of Tagetes minuta', *Journal of Ethnopharmacology*, vol. 56(3), 1997, pp. 227–232.

181 BS Tomova, JS Waterhouse & J Doberski, 'The effect of fractionated Tagetes oil volatiles on aphid reproduction, *Entomologia Experimentalis et Applicata*, vol. 115(1), 2005, pp. 153–159.

182 MJ Perich, C Wells, W Bertsch & KE Tredway, 'Isolation of the insecticidal components of Tagetes minuta (Compositae) against mosquito larvae and adults', *Journal of the American Mosquito Control Association-Mosquito News*, vol. 11(3), 1995, pp. 307–310.

183 L Braun & M Cohen, *Herbs & natural supplements an evidence-based guide volume 2*, 4th edition, Churchill Livingstone (Elsevier), 2014, pp. 933–951.

184 U Quattrocchi, *CRC world dictionary of medicinal and poisonous plants: Common names, scientific names, eponyms, synonyms, and etymology*, CRC Press, Boca Raton, FLA, 2012.

185 Z Stojanović-Radić, L Čomić, N Radulović et al., 'Chemical composition and antimicrobial activity of Erodium species: E. ciconium L., E. cicutarium L., and E. absinthoides Willd. (Geraniaceae)' *Chemical Papers*, vol. 64(3), 2010.

186 MT Lis-Balchin & SL Hart, 'A Pharmacological Appraisal of the Folk Medicinal Usage of Pelargonium grossularioides and Erodium cicutarium', *Journal of Herbs, Spices & Medicinal Plants*, vol. 2(3), 1994, pp. 41–48.

187 D Hornero-Méndez & MI Mínguez-Mosquera, 'Carotenoid pigments in Rosa mosqueta hips, an alternative carotenoid source for foods. Journal of agricultural and food chemistry', vol. 48(3), 2000, pp. 825–828.

188 A Adamczak, W Buchwald, J Zieliński & S Mielcarek, 'Flavonoid and Organic Acid Content in Rose Hips (Rosa L., Sect. Caninae Dc. Em. Christ.)', *Acta Biologica Cracoviensia. Series Botanica*, vol. 54(1), 2012.

189 M Stuart, *The Encyclopedia of Herbs and Herbalism*, Orbis Books, London, 1979, pp. 269–270.

190 CABI Invasive Species Compendium, Tanacetum vulgare (Tansy) www.cabi.org/isc/datasheet/13366.

191 K Pålsson, TG Jaenson, P Baeckström & AK Borg-Karlsonatinka, 'Tick Repellent Substances In The Essential Oil of Tanacetum Vulgare', *Journal of Medical Entomology*, vol. 45.1, 2008, pp. 88–93.

192 Y Aniya, T, Koyama, C Miyagi et al., 'Free radical scavenging and hepatoprotective actions of the medicinal herb, Crassocephalum crepidioides from the Okinawa Islands', *Biological and Pharmaceutical Bulletin*, vol. 28(1), 2005, pp. 19–23.

193 U Quattrocchi, *CRC world dictionary of medicinal and poisonous plants: Common names, scientific names, eponyms, synonyms, and etymology*, CRC Press, Boca Raton, FLA, 2012.

194 CABI Invasive Species Compendium, Datura stramonium (Jimsonweed), www.cabi.org/isc/datasheet/18006.

195 JH Maiden, *The weeds of New South Wales part 1*, Government Printer, Sydney, 1920.

196 A Banso & S Adeyemo, 'Phytochemical screening and antimicrobial assessment of Abutilon mauritianum, Bacopa monnifera and Datura stramonium', *Biokemistri*, vol. 18(1), 2006.

197 P Soni, AA Siddiqui, J Dwivedi & V Soni, 'Pharmacological properties of Datura stramonium L. as a potential medicinal tree: An overview', *Asian Pacific Journal of Tropical Biomedicine*, vol. 2(12), 2012, pp. 1002–1008.

198 Wild Edibles Database http://www.db.weedyconnection.com/plants-a-z/page/5/

199 K Flora, M Hahn, H Rosen & K Benner, 'Milk thistle (Silybum marianum) for the therapy of liver disease', *The American Journal of Gastroenterology*, vol. 93(2), 1998, pp.139–143.

200 F Grases, G Melero, A Costa-Bauzá et al., 'Urolithiasis and phytotherapy', *International Urology and Nephrology*, vol. 26(5), 1994, pp. 507–511.

201 MI Calvo, 'Anti-inflammatory and analgesic activity of the topical preparation of Verbena officinalis L.', *Journal of Ethnopharmacology*, vol. 107(3), 2006, pp.380–382.

202 SG Khattak, SN Gilani & M Ikram, 'Antipyretic studies on some indigenous Pakistani medicinal plants', *Journal of Ethnopharmacology*, vol. 14(1), 1985, pp. 45–51.

203 MH Koochek, MH Pipelzadeh & H Mardani, 'The Effectiveness of Viola odorata in the Prevention and Treatment of Formalin-Induced Lung Damage in the Rat', *Journal of Herbs, Spices & Medicinal Plants*, vol. 10(2), 2003, pp. 95–103.

204 SL Gerlach, R Rathinakumar, G Chakravarty et al., 'Anticancer and chemosensitizing abilities of cycloviolacin O2 from Viola odorata and psyle cyclotides from Psychotria leptothyrsa', *Biopolymers*, vol. 94(5), 2010, pp. 617–625.

205 WH Talib, 'Antiproliferative Activity of Plant Extracts Used Against Cancer In Traditional Medicine', *Scientia Pharmaceutica*, vol. 78(1), 2010, pp. 33–45.

206 DA Kopsell, TC Barickman, CE Sams & JS McElroy, 'Influence of Nitrogen and Sulfur on Biomass Production and Carotenoid and Glucosinolate Concentrations in Watercress

(Nasturtium officinale R. Br.)', *Journal of Agricultural and Food Chemistry*, vol. 55(26), 2007, pp. 10628–10634.

207 T Kaneshiro, M Suzui, R Takamatsu et al., 'Growth inhibitory activities of crude extracts obtained from herbal plants in the Ryukyu Islands on several human colon carcinoma cell lines', *Asian Pacific Journal of Cancer Prevention*, vol. 6(3), 2005, p. 353.

208 DX Tan, LC Manchester, P Di Mascio et al., 'Novel Rhythms of N1-Acetyl-N2-Formyl-5-Methoxykynuramine and Its Precursor Melatonin In Water Hyacinth: Importance For Phytoremediation', *FASEB Journal*, vol. 21(8), 2007, pp. 1724–1729.

209 AM Aboul-Enein, AM Al-Abd, EA Shalaby et al., 'Eichhornia Crassipes (Mart) Solms: From water parasite to potential medicinal remedy', *Plant Signaling & Behavior*, vol. 6(6), 2011, pp. 834–836.

210 J-J Chu, Y Ding & Q-J Zhuang, 'Invasion and Control of Water Hyacinth (Eichhornia Crassipes) In China', *Journal of Zhejiang University. Science. B*, vol. 7(8), 2006, pp. 623–626.

211 F Benencia, MC Courrèges, CE Coto & C Félix, 'Immunomodulatory Activities of Melia Azedarach L. Leaf Extracts On Human Monocytes', *Journal of Herbs, Spices & Medicinal Plants*, vol. 5(3), 1998, pp. 7–13.

212 GM Andrei, CE Coto & RA DeTorres, 'Assays of cytotoxicity and antiviral activity of crude and semipurified extracts of green leaves of Melia azedarach L.', *Revista Argentina de Microbiologia*, vol. 17, 1985, pp. 187–94.

213 PB Oelrichs, MW Hill & PJ Vallely, 'The chemistry and pathology of meliatoxins A and B constituents from the fruit of Melia azedarach Var. Australasica', in *Plant Toxicology: Proceedings of the Australia-USA Poisonous Plant Symposium, Brisbane Australia, May 14–18, 1984*, pp. 387–394.

214 M Roberts, *Indigenous healing plant*, Southern Book Publishers, Cape Town, 1990, pp. 128–129.

215 RB Mulaudzi, AR Ndhlala & J Van Staden, 'Ethnopharmacological evaluation of a traditional herbal remedy used to treat gonorrhoea in Limpopo province, South Africa', *South African Journal of Botany*, vol. 97, 2015, pp. 117–122.

216 E Green, A Samie, CL Obi et al., 'Inhibitory properties of selected South African medicinal plants against Mycobacterium tuberculosis', *Journal of Ethnopharmacology*, vol. 30(1), 2010, pp. 151–157.

217 CAB International Invasive Species Compendium Raphanus raphanistrum (wild radish) www.cabi.org/isc/datasheet/46795.

218 R Jbilou, A Ennabili & F Sayah, 'Insecticidal activity of four medicinal plant extracts against Tribolium castaneum (Herbst)(Coleoptera: Tenebrionidae)', *African Journal of Biotechnology*, vol. 5(10), 2006.

219 F Conforti, S Sosa, M Marrelli et al., 'In vivo anti-inflammatory and in vitro antioxidant activities of Mediterranean dietary plants', *Journal of Ethnopharmacology*, vol. 116(1), 2008, pp. 144–151.

220 U Quattrocchi, *CRC world dictionary of medicinal and poisonous plants: Common names, scientific names, eponyms, synonyms, and etymology*, CRC Press, Boca Raton, FLA, 2012, p. 2728.

221 MP Raghavendra, S Satish & KA Raveesha, 'Phytochemical analysis and antibacterial activity of Oxalis corniculata; a known medicinal plant', *Myscience*, vol. 1(1), 2006, pp. 72–78.

222 PA Abhilash, P Nisha, A Prathapan et al., 'Cardioprotective effects of aqueous extract of Oxalis corniculata in experimental myocardial infarction', *Experimental and Toxicologic Pathology*, vol. 63(6), 2011, pp. 535–540.

223 KJ Achola, JW Mwangi & RW Munenge, 'Pharmacological Activity of Oxalis corniculata', *Pharmaceutical Biology*, vol. 33(3), 1995, pp. 247–249.

224 RF Chandler, SN Hooper & MJ Harvey, 'Ethnobotany and phytochemistry of yarrow, Achillea millefolium, compositae', *Economic Botany*, vol. 36(2), 1982, pp. 203–223.

225 G Innocenti, E Vegeto, S Dall'Acqua et al., 'In vitro estrogenic activity of Achillea millefolium L.', *Phytomedicine*, vol. 14(2–3), 2007, pp. 147–152.

226 A Yildirim, A Mavi & AA Kara, 'Determination of antioxidant and antimicrobial activities of Rumex crispus L. extracts', *Journal of agricultural and food chemistry*, vol. 49(8), 2001, pp. 4083–4089.

227 R Reig, P Sanz, C Blanche et al., 'Fatal poisoning by Rumex crispus (curled dock): pathological findings and application of scanning electron microscopy', *Veterinary and human toxicology*, vol. 32(5), 1990, pp. 468–470.

Bibliography

Auld, BA & Medd, RW, *Weeds: an illustrated botanical guide to the weeds of Australia*, Inkata Press, Melbourne, 1987.

Bone, K & Mills S, *Principles and practice of phytotherapy: moden herbal medicine*, 2nd ed., Churchill Livingstone (Elsevier), 2013.

Braun, L & Cohen, M, *Herbs & natural supplements an evidence-based guide* volume 2, 4th edition, Churchill Livingstone (Elsevier), 2014.

British Herbal Medicine Association, *British Herbal Pharmacopoeia*, UK, 1989.

Collins, P, *Useful seeds at our doorstep (In touch with the Earth)*, Pat Collins, NSW, 1998.

Cowper, AB, Common medicinal plants of Australia, Rose Print, Sydney, 1987.

Ermert, S, *Gardener's companion to weeds*, 2nd ed., New Holland, Sydney, 2001.

Grieve, Mrs M, *A modern herbal*, Tiger Books International, London, 1992. (First published in 1931 by Jonathan Cape Ltd)

Grubb, A & Raser-Rowland, A, *The weed forager's handbook: A guide to edible and medicinal weeds in Australia*, Hyland House Publishing, Australia, 2012.

Hoffman, D, *The new holistic herbal: The bestselling herbal*, Element Publishing, MA, 1983.

Low, T, *Wild herbs of Australia and New Zealand*, Angus & Robertson, Sydney, 1991.

Maiden, JH, *The weeds of New South Wales* part 1, Government Printer, Sydney, 1920.

McCaman, JL, *Weeds and why they grow*, Jay L McCaman, 1994.

Pengelly, A, *Australian Wild Herb Bulletin*, NSW, Australia.

Pfeiffer, EE, *Weeds and what they tell us*, Floris Books, USA, 2012.

Quattrocchi, U, *CRC world dictionary of medicinal and poisonous plants: Common names, scientific names, eponyms, synonyms, and etymology*, CRC Press, Boca Raton, FLA, 2012.

Roberts, M, *Indigenous healing plant*, Southern Book Publishers, Cape Town, 1990.

Stern G, *Australian weeds: A source of natural food and medicine*, Harper & Row, Sydney 1986.

Stuart, M (ed.), *The encyclopedia of herbs and herbalism*, Orbis Books, London, 1979.

van Wyk, B-E & Wink, M, *Medicinal plants of the world*, Timber Press, London, 2004.

Whitten, G, *Herbal harvest: commercial production of quality dried herbs in Australia*, Agmedia, East Melbourne, 1997.

Atlas of Living Australia (www.ala.org.au)
Australian Tropical Rainforest (www.anbg.gov.au)
CABI (www.cabi.org)
Herbal Extract (www.herbalextracts.com.au)
HerbiGuide (www.herbiguide.com.au)
Lucid Fact sheet Fusion (www.lucidcentral.org)
Mediherb (www.mediherb.com.au)
Plants for a Future (www.pfaf.org)
Raintree, Tropical Plant Database (www.rain-tree.com)

Index

Agapanthus	14	Fumitory	88	Prickly Pear	166
Amaranth	16	Golden Rod	90	Purslane	168
Angled Onion	20	Hawthorn	92	Red Flowering Mallow	170
Bathurst Burr	22	Heartsease	94	Saffron Thistle	172
Billygoat Weed	24	Hedge Mustard	96	Salsify	174
Black Thistle	26	Henbit	98	Scarlet Pimpernel	176
Blackberry	28	Honey Locust	100	Self Heal	178
Blackberry Nightshade	30	Honeysuckle, Japanese	104	Sheep Sorrel	180
Bishop's Weed	32	Horehound	106	Shepherd's Purse	182
Borage	34	Inkweed	108	Slender Celery	184
Boxthorn	36	Italian Thistle	110	Sow Thistle	186
Bracken	38	Jasmine	112	Speedwell, Creeping	190
Brassica	40	Jerusalem Artichoke	114	Spiny Emex	192
Bugle	44	Knotweed	116	Stagger Weed	194
Bulrush	46	Lantana	118	Stinking Roger	196
Burdock	48	Lemon Balm	120	St. John's Wort	198
Busy Lizzie	50	Lucerne	122	Storksbill	200
Californian Poppy	52	Mallow	124	Sweet Briar	202
Caltrop	54	Mugwort, Chinese	126	Tansy	204
Centaury	56	Mullein	128	Thickhead	206
Chickweed	58	Nasturtium	132	Thornapple	208
Chicory	60	Nettles	134	Variegated Thistle	212
Clivers	62	Noogoora Burr	138	Vervain	214
Clover	64	Nutgrass	140	Violet, Sweet	216
Cobbler's Pegs	66	Oyster Plant	142	Wandering Jew	218
Dandelion	68	Paddy's Lucerne	144	Watercress	220
Elderberry	70	Pellitory	146	Water Hyacinth	222
English Daisy	72	Pennywort	148	White Cedar	224
False Dandelion	74	Peppercorn Tree	150	Wild Cotton	226
Fat Hen	76	Periwinkle	152	Wild Radish	228
Fennel	78	Petty Spurge	154	Wood Sorrel	230
Feverfew	80	Plantain	156	Yarrow	232
Fishbone Fern	82	Poppy Smallflower Opium	160	Yellow Dock	234
Fleabane	84	Potato Weed	162		
Four O'clock	86	Prickly Lettuce	164		

Index of scientific names

Acanthus mollis	142	
Achillea millefolium	232	
Agapanthus praecox subs. orientalis	14	
Ageratum conyzoides	24	
Ageratum houstonianum	24	
Ajuga reptans	44	
Allium triquetrum	20	
Amaranthus retroflexus	16	
Amaranthus viridis	16	
Ammi majus	26	
Anagallis arvensis	176	
Apium leptophyllum	184	
Arctium lappa	48	
Artemisia verlotorum	126	
Bellis perennis	72	
Bidens pilosa	66	
Borago officinalis	34	
Capsella bursa-pastoris	182	
Carduus pycnocephalus	110	
Carthamus lanatus	172	
Centaurium erythraea	56	
Centaurium spicatum	56	
Centella asiatica	148	
Chenopodium album	76	
Chrysanthemum parthenium/		
Tanacetum parthenium L.	80	
Cichorium intybus	60	
Cirsium vulgare	28	
Conyza bonariensis	84	
Crassocephalum crepidioide	206	
Crataegus monogyna/		
Crataegus laevigata	92	
Cyperus rotundas	140	
Datura stramonium	208	
Eichhornia crassipes	222	
Emex australis	192	
Erodium cicutarium,		
Erodium moschatum	200	
Eschscholzia californica	52	
Euphorbia peplus	154
Foeniculum vulgare	78
Fumaria muralis	88
Galinsoga parviflora	162
Galium aparine	62
Gleditsia triacanthos	100
Gomphocarpus fruticosus/	
Asclepias fruticosa	226
Helianthus tuberosus	114
Hypericum perforatum	198
Hypochoeris radicata	74
Impatiens walleriana	50
Jasminum polyanthum	112
Lactuca serriola	164
Lamium amplexicaule	98
Lantana camara	118
Lonicera japonica	104
Lycium ferocissimum	36
Malva parviflora	124
Marrubium vulgare	106
Medicago sativa	122
Melia azedarach (M. australasica)	224
Melissa officinalis	120
Mirabilis jalapa	86
Modiola caroliniana	170
Nephrolepis cordifolia	82
Opuntia stricta	166
Oxalis corniculata	230
Papaver somniferum ssp. setigerum	160
Perictaria juduica	146
Phytolacca octandra	108
Plantago lanceolata,	
Plantago major	156
Pleridium esculentum,	
Pleridium aquilinum	38
Polygonum aviculare	116
Portulaca oleracea	168
Prunella vulgaris	178
Raphanus raphanistrum	228

Rorippa nasturtiumaquaticum/	
Nasturtium officinale	220
Rosa rubiginosa/	
Rosa arabica Crép/	
Rosa eglanteria L.	202
Rubus fruticosus	30
Rumex acetosella	180
Acetosella vulgaris	180
Rumex crispus	234
Sambucus nigra	70
Schinus molle	150
Sida rhombifolia	144
Silybum marianum	212
Sisymbrium officinale	96
Solanum nigrum	32
Solidago canadensis var. scabra	90
Sonchus oleraceus	186
Stachys arvensis	194
Stellaria media	58
Tagetes minuta	196
Tanacetum vulgare	204
Taraxacum officinale	68
Tradescantia fluminensis (albiflora),	
Commelina cyanea	218
Tragopogon porrifolius	174
Tribulus terrestris	54
Trifolium repens	64
Tropaeolum majus	132
Typha orientalis	46
Typha domingensis	46
Typha latifolia	46
Verbascum thapsus L.	128
Verbena officinalis	214
Veronica persica	190
Vinca major	152
Viola odorata	216
Viola tricolor	94
Xanthium occidentale	138
Xanthium spinosum	22

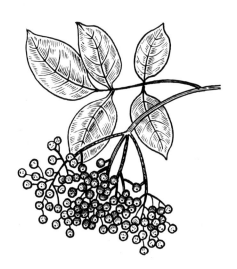